SUSTAINABLE BEAUTY

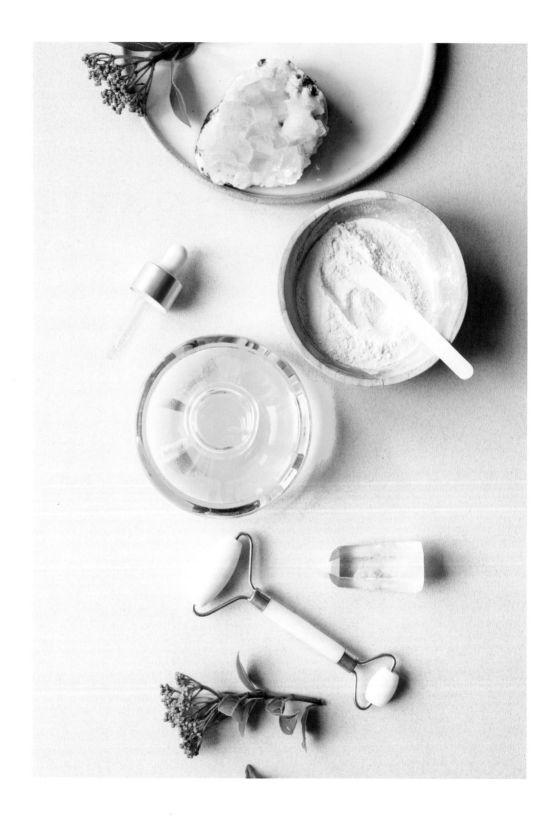

SUSTAINABLE BEAUTY

Practical advice and projects for
an eco-conscious beauty routine

JUSTINE JENKINS

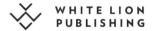
WHITE LION
PUBLISHING

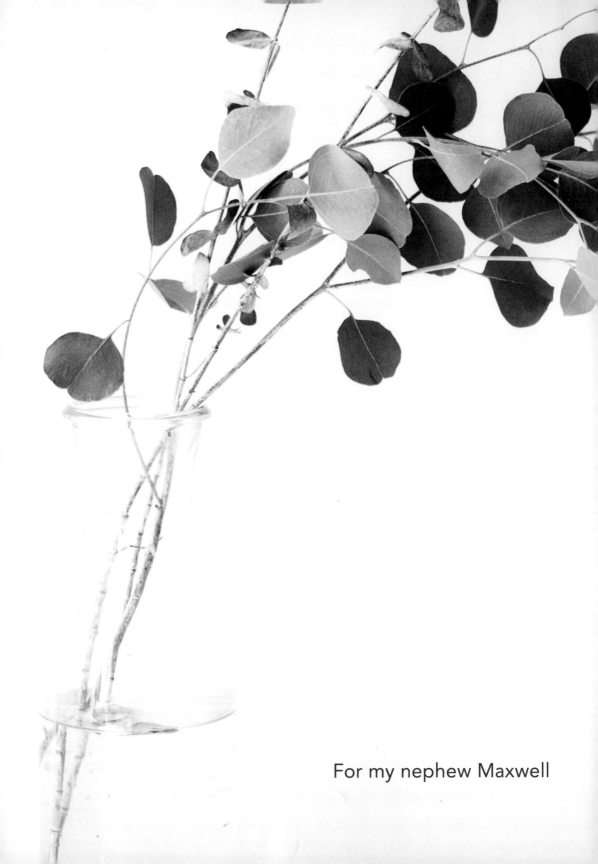

For my nephew Maxwell

Contents

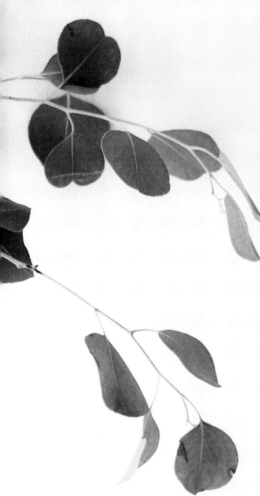

6   Introduction

11 Conscious consumption

15   Defining sustainable beauty
17   What's in a label?
23   The ethical buyer
28   Vegan and vegetarian beauty

31 Our beautiful planet

32   Recyclable, biodegradable and compostable:
     the differences
38   Repurposing your packaging

41 The sustainable self

42   Natural and organic
44   Creating sustainable beauty
48   Skincare
73   Bodycare
90   Haircare

111 Mindful make-up

115   Face
126   Eyes
137   Lips
142   The mindful make-up tool kit
146   Beauty larder
148   Beauty tool shed

150   Conclusion
154   Animal derived ingredients
156   Index
158   Acknowledgements

Introduction

—

Beauty is not just blooming, it's positively booming. In 2019 alone, the industry was valued at a colossal $380.2 billion and is projected to reach $463.5 billion by 2024. But such acceleration of production and voracious consumption must surely call for consideration? It's time to put the brakes on and ask a stark question: at what cost?

I've been a professional make-up artist for 23 years and I *love* my career. The beauty industry is creative, rewarding, bright and beguiling. It's also one of the most unsustainable industries on the planet. In 2012, I was the first prominent make-up artist in London to go entirely cruelty-free after I discovered that most cosmetic brands were *still* testing on animals. Despite brand messaging, a clever and cunning deployment of silky words was misleading the consumer. I decided to speak out. I contacted animal rights charities and organisations to gather the facts and find out what I could do. My mantra became 'If you don't stand for something, you'll fall for everything.' So, I stood up.

Suddenly about 85 per cent of brands – big, global brands – were off my ethical radar. It was not easy. Over the next few years, I wrote hundreds of articles on the subject. The Body Shop invited me to present a petition to the EU in Brussels calling for a global ban of cosmetic animal testing. I visited alternative testing facilities and organic farms that provide ingredients for the beauty industry. Lectures and appearances on panels and podcasts cemented my name as an industry voice. In 2013, I had the privilege of being appointed ambassador for Humane Society International's #BeCrueltyFree campaign. It thrills me that cruelty-free beauty is now mainstream. Oh, and I (might) have got into trouble for sometimes calling out brands for greenwashing!

Animal welfare and natural beauty will always be values at my very core, so that's where I initially focused my efforts. Then, a few years ago, I saw an image that had been posted on Instagram, which forced me to expand both my vision and message.

You too may recall it. A tiny coral-coloured sea horse with its delicate coil of tail wrapped around a plastic cotton bud. There are many images that reveal and poignantly capture the price of our consumption and waste. But that image showed beauty industry waste. My industry. I had used thousands of those little cotton sticks over the years through the course of work. The beauty industry is my problem, but I also believe it's *our* problem. Early on I realised that brands were not doing anything near enough to mitigate or reduce their waste and carbon emissions or improve their manufacturing processes. My eyes were awakened to global deforestation, child labour and farmers barely being able to feed their families. I found myself embarrassed by some elements of my industry, appalled by others. $380 billion dollars, yet we can't be sustainable?

Change cannot happen overnight. I believe in a healthy and vibrant industry – brimming with kaleidoscopic colour, all abilities and breadth of choice for all skin types and tones. Growth and sustainability can go hand in hand, but it will rely on brands building these values into the core of their business. The consumer needs to demand transparency so they can make informed choices and speak with their wallets. Whether you are a consumer, a brand, a make-up artist or an industry professional, will you join me in creating a better, brighter future for beauty? I have spent the past four years researching, the fruit of which is this book – my contribution towards a solution. I share my knowledge and passion from over two decades in the industry, and my journey as a make-up artist, activist, beauty expert and industry reformer. I hope this book is a useful, illuminating and enjoyable read – a treatise, if you like, on how to make beauty sustainable, but also on the enduring and empowering magic of make-up as a conduit for confidence and self-esteem. Behind both constructs are simple forces – love, compassion and care: love of yourself; compassion for animals and the planet; and care of both. I'll guide you through the current issues within the beauty industry, why it needs to change, and how we can make that happen together. I'll encourage you to take a breath and enjoy the ritual of slow beauty, a more conscious, edited, mindful approach. I'll explain how to use less products, to create your own list of essentials, and to enjoy the simplicity of a uncluttered, calm routine.

There's one thing I demand from you though: please eradicate one word from your vocabulary and expunge it from your mind – guilt. It's a waste of time and a drain of power. When we know better, we do better. It starts simply, with one good intention. From a sustainable perspective, everything you do, despite seemingly insignificant, is a powerful positive move. We know when we are doing right, because doing right feels good. We just need to keep building on that.

Finally, I fervently encourage you to use this book. And I mean really use it. Be bold – underline, highlight, fold corners, tag it – do whatever you need to do to learn, expand, grow, be inspired, or get angry! After all, when deployed wisely, anger always converts into action. I look forward to hearing your thoughts, suggestions, ideas and visions through my Instagram @justinejenkins. This is a shared journey and I look forward to treading the trail with you into sustainable beauty for the preservation of our planet. Enjoy it.

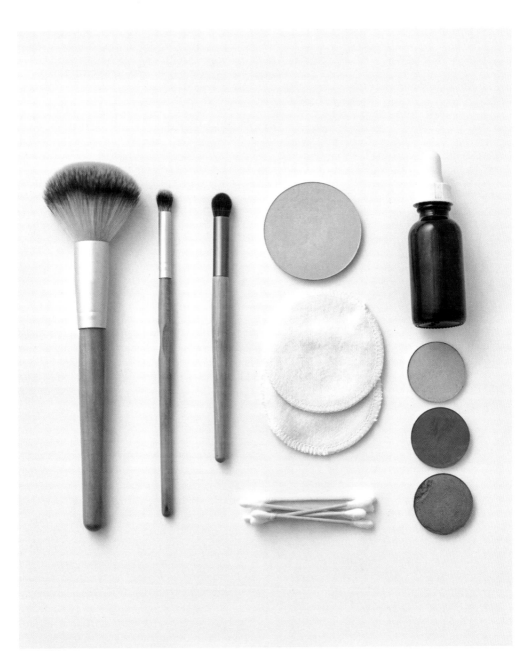

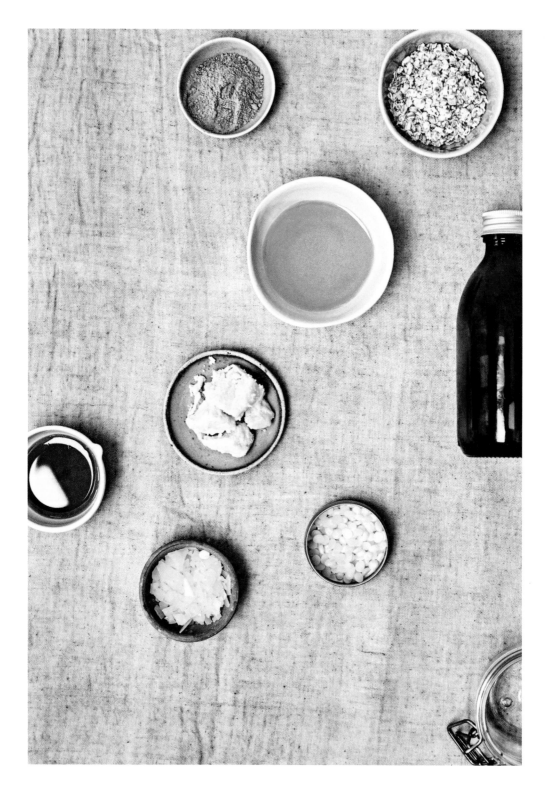

Conscious consumption

—

Never has the consumer (in developed countries) had such plenty, such spectacular array and such exhaustive choice of beauty products. The modern marketplace is global and has been mobbed with all things shiny. No longer are beauty products deemed a luxury by people of any generation, race or gender, but rather a necessity. Yet how many consumers are able to make ethical, informed buying choices?

Marketing can morph into many forms. It shapeshifts from the obvious advertisement, to discreet brand marketing across a spectrum of social media platforms, to a vlogger, blogger, influencer, or online tutorial, a #paidpartnership an #ad posted by a 'blue-tick' we follow on Instagram.

For much of the time we don't even realise that we are being marketed to. Creeping like long summer shadows, ads are under our noses and before we even know it, their covert code has been absorbed and decrypted. Deciphered by the brain and projected as desires (or fears), triggering the 'INT' (I *need* that) response, just as we find a rogue thumb twitching over 'add to cart'. And we're even barely conscious of just how we got there. But we've all been there, haven't we?!

Studies show that consumers spend less time considering their purchases than ever before. It's just so easy to swipe, tap, and chip. Tech, tablets and phones, have gifted the shopper 24-hour accessibility to retail therapy. I'm not sure that this situation as it stands offers a happy outcome when you think in terms of global impact and what that *really* means.

However, I believe there has been a shift in global conscience. Consumers are demanding more transparency from brands. They want to know what impact their buying choices will have on their environment. While the rush to become more eco-friendly has only really taken hold in the last five years or so – and long may it continue – the journey to becoming a truly conscious beauty consumer can be bewildering, full of confusion and misinformation. How do we avoid 'greenwashing', how can we be more sustainable, and how do we reduce our beauty consumption without compromising on the health of our skin, hair and love of make-up in a world in which beauty matters?

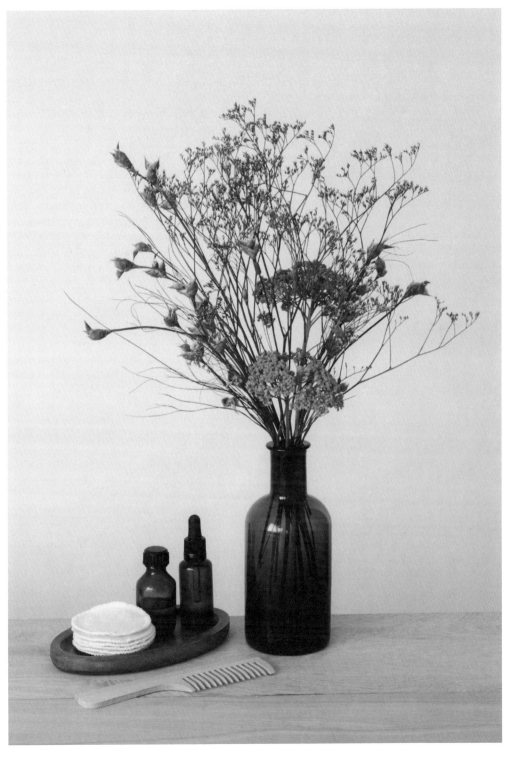

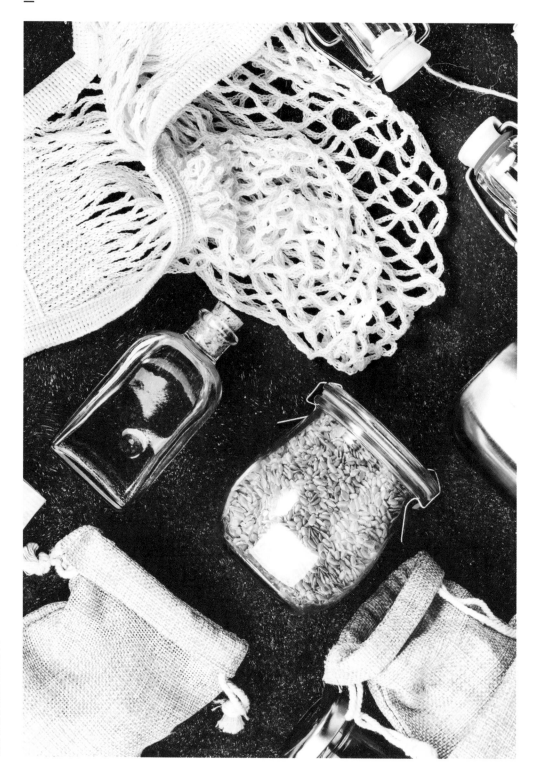

Defining sustainable beauty

—

As much as we may adore our beauty products, the 'lion's share' of the wider industry is anything but sustainable; that world-weary word means more than most realise. Sustainability is a system that maintains its own viability by using techniques that allow for continual reuse, a circular journey – if you like. This phrase 'continual reuse' is the key. For too long we have been led as a society to consume without thought or conscience. This has a cost to our wallet, and crucially, to the environment.

I believe that there is good news. If we take positive steps now – we can turn this around. The voice of the consumer is a powerful one. It speaks a universal and widely understood language. The language is called cash! It's easy to think we are just individuals and our independent choices have no impact, but even one small change has a ripple effect, and if there are more people like us, those ripples eventually turn into waves. So, if we apply a more edited approach to beauty consumption, purchasing more ethically minded and sustainable brands, we can have an impact on the way the industry develops.

Sustainable beauty means different things to different people, so it really boils down to what is important to you. Issues you may want to consider are: human and animal welfare, employee diversity, the amount of miles ingredients and final products have travelled, damage to biodiversity and to the environment, carbon and water footprint, the quality of ingredients and how they are grown, renewable resources, aquatic damage, waste management and unsustainable packaging materials.

As you can see, there is much to consider behind the glitz and glamour. Some of these issues will touch a nerve within you, whilst others won't feel so important right now. It's impossible to tick all those boxes, so start with one. Research the brands you use, and get informed. Brands that have true sustainability at their core, will be able to answer your questions. We won't always make perfect choices, but we can strive to do what we can. This book will serve you as a sustainable beauty guide. And, if we change our attitude towards consumption, we can make this sustainable beauty journey a positive and successful one.

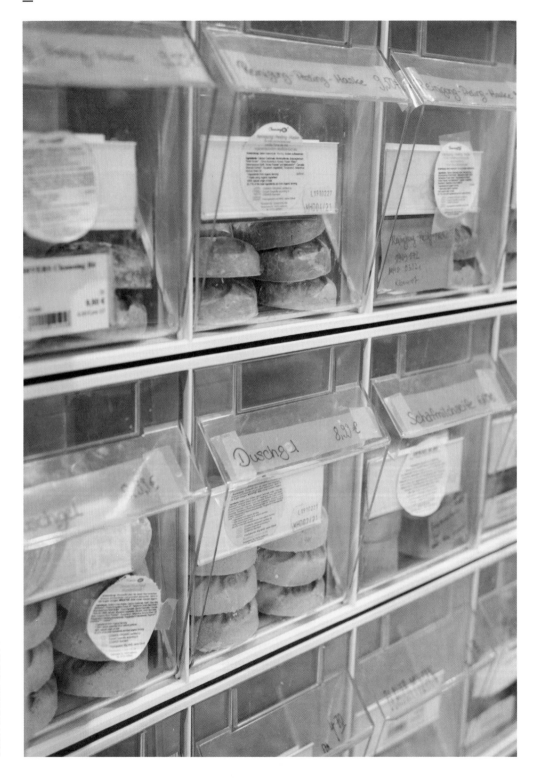

What's in a label?

—

Being able to read a label and know exactly what's in, and what's not in a product, is empowering. In an instant, we can check the label and know that what we are buying is exactly what we are looking for. If it contains ingredients we are sensitive to, if it's certified cruelty-free, vegan, organic, or if it's plastic-free. But is it as easy as it sounds?

The International Nomenclature of Cosmetic Ingredients, or INCI list, is, for us lay folk, the ingredients list. The ingredients included in the product in the highest quantities are at the top of the list, and descends in order of concentration. One of the difficulties in reading the INCI list, is that the ingredients are often listed with just their chemical name or, for plant extracts, their Latin name, so how do we know what they are? I've listed some common ingredients (see pages 20–21) but grab a copy of *Milady's Skin Care and Cosmetics Ingredients Dictionary* if you want to delve deeper. That book is my bible. Other details to consider are where the ingredient originated, and whether it is vegetable or animal derived. This is especially confusing if you want to purchase locally grown ingredients, or vegan products, for example.

Certifications

One way to ensure what you are buying truly aligns with issues that are important to you, is to check on the label for certifications. Any brand can legally state their products are natural, cruelty-free or organic when they're not, so a certified product removes any confusion. If a product shows the Soil Association or Cosmos symbol, you know it's certified organic. If it bears the Fair Trade logo, you know it's a high quality, ethically produced product. If it has the Vegan Society trademark, you know it's vegan. If it bears the logo for Leaping Bunny (CFI, non-US and Canadian), CCIC Leaping Bunny (US and Canada), Choose Cruelty Free (CCF, Australia) or PETA symbol, you know it's cruelty free. If the brand is B Corp certified then you know it meets the highest standard of social and environmental performance. Stick to the tried and tested certifications, and be aware of symbols and logos that mean nothing. Many of them do not have any merit, so you will need to research their legitimacy. Licensing the symbols used on packaging, comes at a cost to the brand, so the absence of a symbol doesn't automatically mean the product isn't what it says it is. Don't be afraid to ask brands questions. You'll soon develop an understanding of their ethos and decide if they are right for you.

Terminology

Do you know your 'nontoxic' from your 'non-GMO', or the difference between 'organic' and 'biodynamic'? Different terminologies are used to define a sustainable beauty product. It's confusing, so I've highlighted some common terms you may read about, or see on packaging.

Alcohol-free
This refers to fermented alcohols, which dry the skin and hair. Products including long-chain fatty alcohols can still be labelled 'alcohol-free'.

Anhydrous
This means 'water-less'. People choose water-less products for reasons including less need for separate preservatives, and water scarcity. There is still a water footprint somewhere, so many prefer the term 'water responsible.' This includes reducing water usage in growing ingredients, manufacturing and shipping products and washing packaging for recycling.

Biodynamic skincare
Described as 'organic plus', biodynamic ingredients are grown holistically, without harmful chemicals, and according to the lunar cycle. The principle is that the efficacy of the product is directly related to the quality of the soil and the ingredients grown. Certification body is Demeter.

Blue beauty
Brands that have a net positive impact on the environment. Green beauty focuses on having a better impact on the environment, whereas blue beauty brands go one step further by giving back and improving the environment.

Carbon neutral
The amount of carbon dioxide or other carbon compounds (CO_2 emissions) generated during the product's life cycle are reduced to zero as they are offset by actions to balance them. Brands use charitable organisations to plant trees.

CBD skincare
CBD is a cannabinoid derived from the cannabis plant. When CBD reacts with the receptors in our body, they have a positive effect on skin health. As powerful antioxidants, they can slow down the ageing process; as anti-inflammatories they are excellent for acne and sensitive skin, and their soothing properties calm down reactive skin.

Chemical-free
Technically, there is no such thing as 'chemical-free' as all matter is chemical, even water. It's used as more of an umbrella term by brands referring to harsher synthetic chemicals, so customers immediately know the products are more natural.

Circular Beauty
Brands that utilise a manufacturing process where waste is eliminated, and resources continually used.

Clean beauty
Used to describe products that concentrate on well being. They are natural based, and less likely to include ingredients that cause skin to react. It's a term also used to describe brands that are transparent in their marketing material.

Cruelty-Free
A product that has not been tested on animals during any part of its manufacture, and does not sell in any territories that requires animal testing.

Green beauty
There is no global definition, but generally green beauty products contain ingredients from nature, and are manufactured to reduce environmental damage. It also incorporates social causes. 'Green washing' describes brands not as green as they say they are.

Hypoallergenic
Products that avoid ingredients likely to cause sensitivities.

Microbiome skincare

Our microbiome is made up of trillions of bacteria, fungi and microbes in our bodies, including our skin. Microbiome skincare means the product is doesn't over-sanitise the skin or cause an imbalance to the microbiome.

Natural skincare

There is no set industry standard to the term 'natural' in beauty products. Natural ingredients can be raw natural ingredients and they can also be heavily processed in a lab, or mixed with synthetic ingredients.

Non-comedogenic

An ingredient that is less likely to block pores and cause a whitehead, blackhead or blemish (comedone).

Non-GMO

The FDA considers genetically modified organisms (GMO) safe. Greenpeace, argue their risks have not been adequately identified. Many brands remove these ingredients from their products altogether.

Nontoxic

This is an umbrella term to describe products that eliminate certain ingredients that are questionable to our health. It's important to understand that toxicity has different variables, including dosage and delivery system. All ingredients used in our cosmetics have been deemed safe by scientists, but many question their long term usage.

Organic

In the beauty industry, the term 'organic' is currently an unregulated claim. Some products indicate the percentage of organic ingredients on the label, which can vary from product to product, and can be as little as 1%.

Paraben-free

All products need a preservation system to prevent microbial and bacterial contamination. The use of parabens in cosmetics became controversial after a 2004 UK study stated that they are bioaccumulative (have continuous build-up) and linked to breast cancers. This study has since been debunked, but the popularity of paraben-free products indicates that consumers want more information on their long-term use.

Skinimilism

A concept of using only what you need. What beauty products are essential to you, and what can you eliminate?

Slow beauty

An attitude to beauty that incorporates mind, body and spirit. It's about choosing quality products aligned to wellbeing for us and for the planet, and making changes that give our beauty routines breathing space, eliminating overwhelm.

Sustainable

This is measured by the process of sourcing the ingredients, the supply chain, the product's packaging, renewable resources, diversity and waste management. Sustainable beauty brands are transparent with this information.

Vegan beauty

A product that does not contain any animal, or animal derived ingredients.

Zero waste

According to Zero Waste Europe, this means 'designing and managing products and processes to reduce the volume and toxicity of waste and materials, conserve and recover all resources and not burn or bury them.'

Ingredients

Each country or territory has a regulatory body who assess the safety of cosmetics sold there. Tens of thousands of ingredients are used in beauty products, all deemed safe in the doses used, but are some of them harmful? The EU has banned or restricted over 1,300 chemicals, while the US has outlawed or curbed just 11. As with all toxins, any risk to health is dependent on many factors including dose and the route by which a substance enters the body. Here are some examples of ingredients that can potentially cause sensitivities, or negative health effects.

Acetone and ethyl acetate

Solvents primarily used in nail polish removers. Both can be very drying and irritating to the skin. Alternatives are milder bio solvents derived from corn, sugar cane and wheat.

AHA and BHA

Alpha hydroxy acid (glycolic and lactic acid) and beta hydroxy acid (salicylic acid) are used to exfoliate skin and improve signs of ageing, dry skin and uneven skin tone. Both can make a positive difference to skin, but moderation is advised. AHA can make your skin sun sensitive, and BHA can cause dryness.

Alcohol

Alcohols are used for antiseptic, antibacterial and antiviral properties. There are two major types of alcohols in beauty products: short-chain alcohols are quick to evaporate, so manufacturers use them in products like hairsprays and toners. In high amounts, they evaporate moisture, causing dryness. People with oily skin like their quick degreasing nature, however stripping away too much natural oil can cause increased oil production. Long-chain fatty alcohols, have a different chemical structure, allowing them to trap water. They can make creams smoother, lotions thicker, and hair hydrated and soft. They're either derived from plants and oils or synthesised in a lab.

Bismuth oxychloride

Used as a make-up colorant, it creates an iridescent effect. Found in products, including mineral cosmetics. It's described as a potential skin irritant, so avoid if you have sensitive skin.

Essential oils

Derived from plants, herbs and flowers, essential oils are in many beauty formulations. They're potent botanicals and should always be diluted. If you have sensitive skin avoid essential oils, as they can cause irritations.

Formaldehyde

Banned in EU beauty products, formaldehyde is still approved for use in the US and Australia. Found in some hair-straightening treatments and nail polish. A known irritant, it can cause watery eyes, coughing and difficulty breathing.

Fragrance

This 'ingredient' can be made up of a few hundred different ingredients. Despite there begin many more, manufacturers are only required to list 26 ingredients if they are present at certain levels, due to them being a common cause of sensitivities. Fragrance is the biggest cause of adverse reactions, so choose 'fragrance-free' products if you have sensitive skin.

Free radicals

Whilst not an ingredient per say, these unstable molecules can cause damage to our skin cells. Caused by air pollution, stress, UV radiation, pesticides, pharmaceutical drugs, industrial chemicals, smoking, alcohol, the food we eat, the water we drink and an unhealthy lifestyle. It's impossible to avoid them entirely, but we can offset their harm by including antioxidants, such as vitamins A, B3, C and E, in our beauty routine.

Oxybenzone

A naturally occurring chemical found in flowering

plants that absorbs UV rays. The Environmental Working Group (EWG) warns consumers to avoid this sunscreen agent, as it can cause allergic reactions. Claims include toxicity to reproductive systems. It infiltrates our oceans through sunscreens worn by swimmers and through our sewage systems. There are claims it bleaches coral reefs creating lasting damage. An in vitro (lab setting) confirmed this, but no conclusive study has yet been done in a marine environment.

Parabens

See Paraben-free

PFAS

A group of synthetic chemicals, used to make products water repellant and stain resistant. Found in products advertised as 'wear-resistant' 'long-lasting' and 'waterproof'. They never break down naturally, and have been found in oceans, local water supplies, in humans and marine life. During 2005–2013, a C8 Science Panel study concluded a probable link between PFAS and high cholesterol, ulcerative colitis, thyroid disease, testicular and kidney cancer.

Phthalates

A group of chemical compounds used to make plastics more flexible. They boost absorption and are also used as solvents. They are in packaging, nail products, hairsprays, deodorant, shampoos and perfume. Where they have been identified as a health hazard, their use has been restricted.

Propellants

Propellants are used to force fluids such as hairsprays, antiperspirants and other aerosol products out of a can. Some have been banned by the FDA due to their potential health hazards.

Silicones

Silicones in products smooth skin, and give dry and damaged hair shine. Over time they may weigh down hair making it dull and brittle. Some don't break down, leaving an environmental impact. Vegetable glycerin is a healthier alternative, and raw apple cider vinegar rinses remove build-up without stripping the hair.

Surfactants

Avoid these ingredients if you have dry skin or coarse, dry, Afro or curly hair. They create foam and lather, neither of which have any benefit, and can cause dryness, redness and irritation. Natural alternatives such as coco glucoside, are gentler and better for your hair and skin, as opposed to synthetic versions like Sodium Lauryl Sulfate.

Talc

Talc, talcum powder or French chalk is a bulking agent also used to absorb moisture and oil. Restricted in the EU, but not in the US. The International Agency for Research on Cancer classifies genital use of talc-based body powder as possibly carcinogenic to humans. Asbestos free talc is considered safe to use in cosmetics.

Toluene

Listed as benzene, methylbenzene, phenylmethane and toluol, and found in hair dyes and nail polishes. The Environmental Working Group (EWG) considers it highly toxic, associated with immune system toxicity and some cancers. The United States Environmental Protection Agency (EPA) believes there is inadequate information to assess its carcinogenic potential.

Triclosan

A synthetic anti-bacterial and antifungal agent and preservative it's restricted in the EU. High dosages may lead to side effects such as abnormal endocrine system and a weakened immune system. A study published in the Journal of Clinical Endocrinology and Metabolism, analysed data from 1,848 women, and found those with higher levels of triclosan in their urine were more likely to have bone issues.

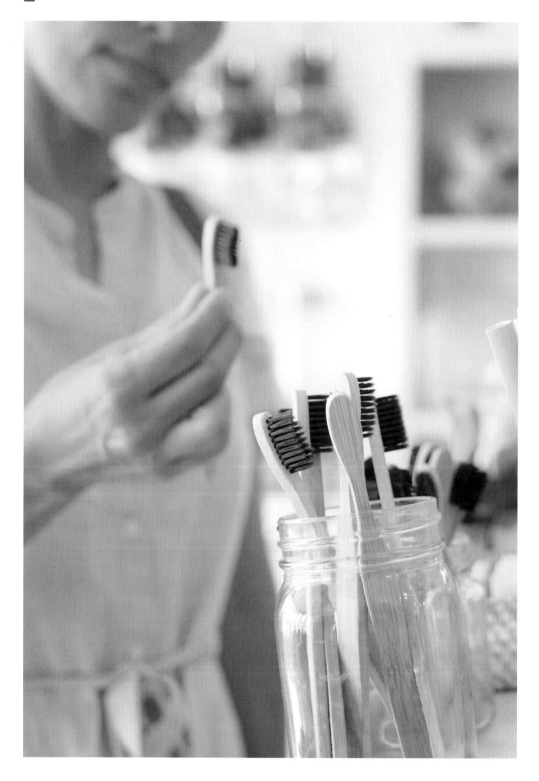

The ethical buyer

—

We can make so many positive changes that will move the beauty industry in a more sustainable direction. I've outlined 9 pillars below, to support you in making that change. I call these pillars S.T.A.R.C.

Spending power – as the consumer, the power is in your hands. Direct your spending to more sustainable brands, and the industry will get the message. Support the brands that care about animals, people and the planet.

Transparency – demand transparency from the brands you buy. Email them and tell them what is important and valuable to you. You have a right to know about their supply chain.

Action – email the brands that put profits over the planet. Ask questions, such as where their manufacturing ingredients are from or if they're conflict-free, use non-GMO ingredients, use child labour, harm animals or contribute to deforestation. If they feel there is a big enough demand, they will change.

Reduce – the biggest impact you can have on sustainability, is to reduce what products you use and buy.

Recycle – get informed about what packaging can be recycled at home in your area, and what needs specialist recycling. If funds allow, invest in a TerraCycle box (www.terracycle.com) for hard to recycle items.

Reuse/Repurpose – even better than recycling, is reusing existing packaging for other purposes.

Refill – choose brands that offer refillable options. Some supermarkets, as well as local shops, now offer this service for beauty products. Carbon conscious companies like Loop, offer refillable products delivered to your door.

Research – don't take as verbatim what companies say on their packaging or website: question them. Brands that have an elevated moral compass will be only too willing to answer.

Create your own – a great way of consuming less. You will have to purchase the ingredients you don't already have, but they'll produce a lot more product for your buck.

CONSCIOUS CONSUMPTION

Sourcing your product

How do we know ingredients are sourced ethically? Fair Trade was set up to prevent the unethical treatment of individuals and the environment to maximise profits. It encourages companies to consider 'building an entire business around a social mission' and it challenges us to confront the systemic exploitation involved in manufacturing and consuming products. By respecting each person in the supply chain, consumers can use purchasing power to evoke change. Many small brands cannot afford Fair Trade certification, but it does not mean they are not ethical. Speak to them and find out their back story.

For too many brands, people, animals and the planet come second to profit. This is why we have to be awakened, start to ask brands the right questions so that the industry is held accountable. Take two of the biggest ingredients in beauty products: mica and palm oil. Mica is mined in India and Madagascar, while most of the world's palm oil derives from Indonesia and Malaysia. I've chosen these ingredients to highlight child labour and global deforestation, as examples of what can occur when we continue to voraciously consume. These are by no means isolated examples, and many more ingredients are grown with the same heavy costs to communities and their environment.

Mica

An ingredient that gives glitter and shimmer to our beauty products, mica has a less sparkling side to it. Child labour is a huge problem within the natural mica mining industry, especially in illegal mines in India and Madagascar. If a brand uses mica from these areas, there is no way of knowing if child labour has been involved. Children as young as five are used because they are small and can easily enter the tiny, narrow mine shafts. Many are injured or die. But as mica is sold on to different intermediaries, it's virtually impossible to trace the source and check if the supply chain is child-labour-free.

So, what can we do? Email and ask brands where they source their mica. If they don't know, avoid them. If we tell them this issue is important to us, it'll matter. You have the power to be a change-maker by allowing your voice to be heard.

Buying mica from regulated territories with anti-child-labour regulations, such as the US or Malaysia, sends this message loud and clear. This dilemma with natural mica is why many brands, even natural and organic ones, choose to use synthetic mica.

Palm oil

You may have seen the Greenpeace footage of terrified Bornean orangutans fighting off the huge diggers destroying their habitat, and the disturbing images of dead orangutans , all in the name of palm oil. Over 80 per cent of their habitat has been annihilated in the last 20 years, and if we do not act now, we may see their extinction in our lifetime. In equal danger, due to palm oil deforestation, are Sumatran elephants, tigers, rhinos and Malaysian sun bears. Environmental damage due to palm oil plantations is so vast that we are witnessing the demise of some of the richest biodiversity that we'll ever see. The UN is calling it a conservation emergency.

Palm oil is found in 70 per cent of beauty products. Why is it so popular? It's the cheapest vegetable oil to produce, and beauty manufacturers love it as it thickens, emulsifies, holds colour and doesn't melt at high temperatures. However, because it is a mass-produced crop, the industry does not look at accountability for environmental and social costs, which are huge. It's estimated that, in Malaysia and Indonesia, an area the size of 300 football fields of virgin rainforest is destroyed every hour to make way for palm oil plantations. Many traditional communities have lost their land to plantations, and human rights abuses, such as child labour, human trafficking and the destruction of indigenous villages, are well documented. Over 50 million metric tonnes of palm oil is produced each year and demand is forecast to double by 2030 and triple by 2050.

Many companies use what is called 'sustainable palm oil', but evidence suggests that the decline in orangutan populations is equal, whether or not a plantation has a sustainable certification. I believe this to be because sustainable palm oil simply means that no further rainforest is destroyed for growth. This is a better option, but it does not reverse the damage already done.

Unbelievably, there is no industry body to determine which companies use sustainable palm oil. Currently, the only certification available to companies is the RSPO (Roundtable on Sustainable Palm Oil). Being a member of the RSPO means a company has committed to eventually use or create sustainable palm oil, but it doesn't mean it is doing so. RSPO members like Unilever, Cadbury's, Nestle and L'Oréal make up 40 per cent of the global palm oil trade.

Many argue that avoiding palm oil is not the answer because other crops use more natural resources including water. Even if we want to, it's sometimes hard to know if palm oil is in a product or not. There are over 200 names for palm oil, so reading the INCI list is often not enough.

So what can we do? Support environmental organisations such as the Orangutan Project, Orangutan Foundation International (OFI) and Rainforest Action Network. Tell major brands you are refusing to purchase them because of their overuse of palm oil, and encourage them to stop using it altogether. Check out the comprehensive list of palm-oil-free companies on www.ethicalconsumer.org, which also lists companies using certified organic palm oil, together with a fully traceable supply chain. Look for the POFCAP logo, which is the international certificate of palm-oil-free brands.

Cruelty-free beauty

I don't think you can pursue a sustainable beauty journey without considering the implications of the beauty industry on animal welfare. Back in 2012, I attended a course on how to make your own natural cosmetics. I've always been inspired by natural beauty, so this course felt like the right step. Headed by a brilliant biochemist, it included various modules. One of which was to prove a revelation; a lesson on how to read product labels and symbols. One symbol jumped out at me, the Leaping Bunny logo, created by the charity Cruelty Free International (CFI). The appearance of this logo on packaging, confirms CFI have verified that product to be cruelty-free, and therefore not tested on animals. I was appalled: I remember going on anti-vivisection marches as a teen, and assumed the beauty industry had stopped animal testing years ago. When I voiced my surprise and disbelief, the biochemist told me to go and research. I did. It was an eye-opener to find animal testing still so prevalent – so much so, that at the time, only a few brands could truly call themselves 'cruelty-free'.

Let me be clear: the term 'cruelty-free', solely refers to animal testing. It does not mean it's vegan, natural, clean or organic.

After discovering the truth, I knew deep in my gut that I had to be a cruelty-free make-up artist. It's a no-brainer: once you've seen the extreme cruelty inflicted on animals, all for the sake of a new mascara or shampoo, there is no going back. It cannot be justified in any way, not even for a miracle formulation to end all our beauty problems. It quickly became apparent that few of my peers were aware that animal testing in our industry still existed. So, if we, as industry professionals, didn't know, then how on earth could the consumer know? It was beauty's ugly secret. I knew I had to spread awareness, talk, write and shout about it, to educate consumers and colleagues as to what they were spending their hard-earned cash on.

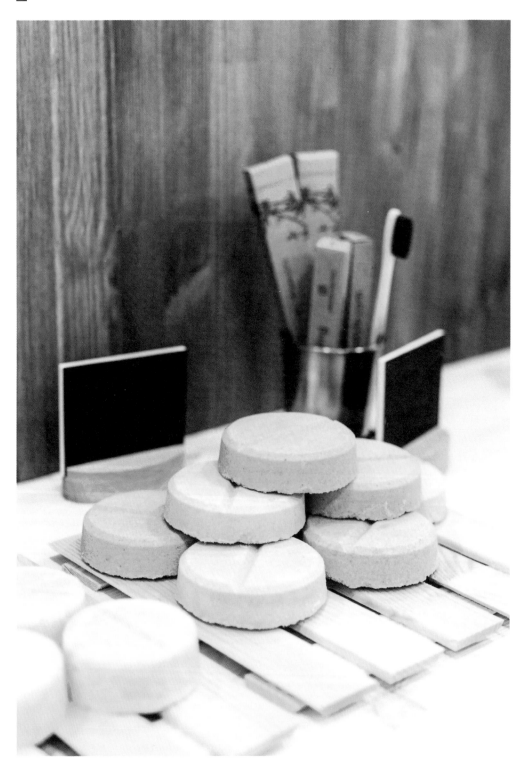

Is this product animal tested?

Why were we all so ignorant? Well, there was a web of clever brand-marketing language covering up the truth. This was abruptly brought home to me when I decided to create my first cruelty-free looks for a red carpet event. I wanted to use two big brands which, on their website, claimed to be cruelty-free. They sent me products; I used them; a magazine wrote a piece on it; job done. I then started delving into their cruelty-free certification, and realised that the brands I had used didn't have any. When I asked why, both brands claimed they didn't have the time or resources to get certified, so I offered my services for free. To say a wall came down was an understatement. They went from sending pleasant emails stating they didn't have the time, to completely ghosting me when I started to ask probing questions. Confused, I contacted animal charity PETA. They explained, 'This is common behaviour, as there is no law to stop a brand saying they are cruelty-free when they are not.' Brands may disguise their true position on animal testing by using confusing language. Here are some examples of the sentences you may come across:

– *This product is not tested on animals* – This statement does not mention ingredients. Therefore, while the final product may be clean of animal testing, the ingredients that make up that product may not be.
– *We don't test on animals unless required by law* – This is a warning that the brand is already selling, or is open to selling, in territories that require animal testing by law.
– *This company does not test on animals* – This may mean the company contracts out its testing to other companies.

So you see how easy it is to be duped. This is why we all need to be aware, in order to force brands to be clear with their marketing language. It's essential that there is transparency, so consumers can make informed choices.

Ethical brands

PETA, Leaping Bunny and Logical Harmony are examples of charities and websites that run their own lists of cruelty-free brands. Each have their own criteria, so check which one you feel comfortable using. I always check for more than one certification; for example, if a brand is PETA-certified, I'll look at CFI or Logical Harmony to make sure it's on their list too. If a brand is small and isn't yet certified, or cannot afford the costs associated with certification, question them directly. If they are proud of being cruelty-free, then they will happily give you all the information you need. If they reply with unclear answers, then alarm bells should start ringing. Here are some questions you may want to ask:

Q: Do you sell in countries that require animal testing by law?
Some countries require cosmetic products sold in their territory to be tested on animals.

Q: Are the ingredients you use tested on animals by you or a third party?
Most historical ingredients have been tested on animals in the past. However, this doesn't mean they can never be a cruelty free ingredient. The manufacturers should supply the brand with a cut off date which denotes when the ingredient stopped being tested on animals, and can be used in cruelty-free formulations.

Q: Are your final products tested by you or a third party?
Even if the brand doesn't test on animals, a government body, for example, may.

Q: Are you happy for this information to be published online?
If a brand is being untruthful about it's animal testing policy, they won't want to draw any attention to the subject of animal testing.

Laws and regulations are constantly changing. For the most up to date information, please go to my blog www.justainablebeauty.com.

Vegan and vegetarian beauty

—

A vegetarian beauty product is one that does not contain any animal ingredients such as shark squalene. A vegan product is one that is vegetarian, but in addition does not contain any animal-derived ingredients, such as milk, beeswax, and honey. To check if a product is vegan, read ingredient labels and look for certified vegan symbols like that of the Vegan Society. In terms of sustainable beauty, there's a big debate about whether a product can be truly cruelty-free if it is not also vegan. For example, the animal cruelty and environmental horrors of the dairy industry are well reported, and large scale beekeeping causes many bees to die. You'll see from the list of popular beauty ingredients on pages 20–21 that we may not fully realise where these ingredients come from. I challenge you not to be at least a little shocked. Then consider, and make an informed decision about whether you want your products to be not only cruelty-free, but vegetarian or vegan too.

That said, don't assume all vegan products are cruelty-free. I'm seeing several large non-cruelty-free brands launching vegan ranges. One would assume that if you don't want animal-derived ingredients in your products, then you also want them free from animal testing. However, veganism is rapidly increasing in popularity and brands want to cash in on that 'trend'. Before buying any vegan products, make sure that brand is also certified cruelty-free.

Another common assumption is that every vegan brand is organic, natural and green. Carmine, for instance, is a red dye that is derived from crushed female cochineal beetles. As it's animal derived and comes from the natural world, it is considered a 'natural' ingredient. However, in a vegan product, carmine would be replaced with a synthetic dye. Many vegan products are of course natural and organic too, but the term itself only refers to whether the ingredients come from an animal.

Other items to be aware of are false eyelashes, which can be made from mink hair and can contain silk. Some brands claim their lashes are made from 'ethically sourced mink hair'. This industry is unregulated, and these animals are farmed and often kept in tiny, dirty cages, without the freedom to move. There is nothing ethical about that. Make-up brushes that are made from 'natural bristles' or 'natural fibres' can include squirrel, horse, fox and sable. Likewise, hairbrushes made from 'natural fibres' are usually made from boar bristle or horse hair. Synthetic brushes are made from non-animal-derived fibres, however it's best to ensure your brushes are also labelled vegan.

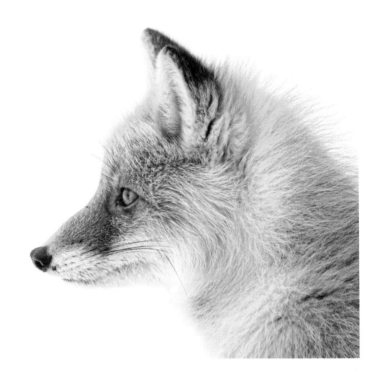

Parent companies

<u>BEAUTY DILEMMA:</u> What about cruelty-free brands that are owned by parent companies that are not cruelty-free?

Many big non cruelty-free brands buy smaller cruelty-free brands and become their parent company. This causes confusion if you want to be cruelty-free and the parent company is not. There are two ways to look at this. One is to only purchase independent cruelty-free brands who have not been bought by another non-cruelty-free company. The other way is to continue to support the brand in their cruelty-free status by informing the parent company that you want them to remain cruelty-free, and stop purchasing them if they become non cruelty-free. Why bother doing this and not just stick to independent brands? Parent companies are usually big corporations, and big business. They could easily take the cruelty-free brand into huge markets where they would no longer be cruelty-free and more animals will suffer. They are less likely to do this, if enough people email them, as they will recognise the demand for the brand to remain cruelty-free. For example, in 2012, cruelty-free brand Urban Decay were purchased by L'Oréal. They then announced plans to sell in countries that required animal testing by law, which would mean they'd no longer be cruelty-free. So many customers complained, that they decided to rescind this decision in order to remain cruelty-free. Whether the initial decision to sell in those countries was theirs, or it was enforced by L'Oréal, no one knows, but what we can see here is the power to change by letting your voice be heard.

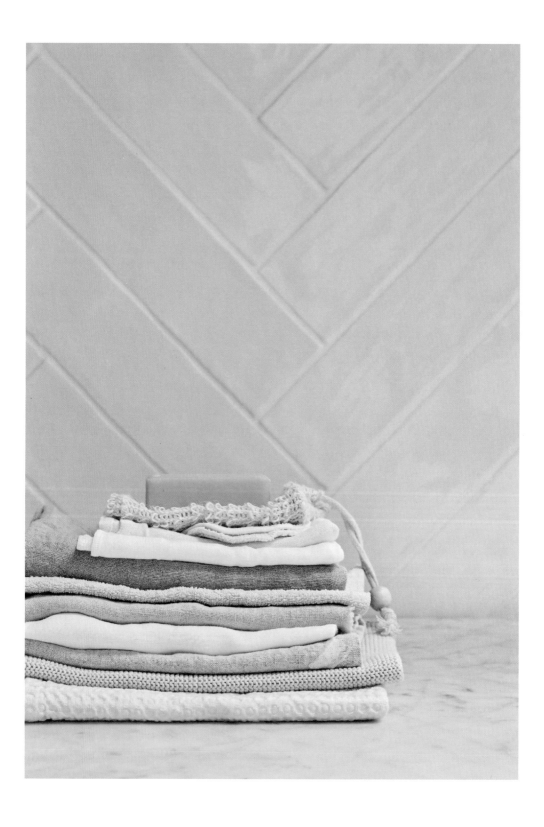

Our beautiful planet

—

The Ellen MacArthur Foundation, a charity that promotes the circular economy, estimates there'll be more plastic than fish in the ocean by 2050. The growth in single-use consumer plastics has fuelled a surge in plastic pollution around the world. It is estimated there are now 5.25 trillion pieces of ocean plastic debris. Shocking, isn't it? Packaging, including beauty packaging, accounts for a whopping 40 per cent of plastic usage. The cosmetic industry alone creates 120 billion pieces of packaging every single year and takes up a third of all landfill space. The fact is that most cosmetic packaging is unrecyclable in your curbside bin. We need brands to step up in two ways: use more packaging that is simple and easy to recycle, and to give the consumer more transparent information on how to recycle their packaging.

In 2020, I was invited by a great cruelty-free, vegan brand to collaborate on a product. When it came to the packaging, I knew I wanted a fully recycled and recyclable product that was plastic-free. However, every avenue I went down, was met with an obstacle, and every packaging manufacturer I contacted, couldn't supply it. This packaging just didn't exist. In the end, we postponed the project as I wasn't happy compromising. Beauty packaging was not my area of expertise, but I wanted to learn more, so I started a personal research project to understand exactly what beauty products could be recycled, how and where (see pages 32–37).

Recyclable, biodegradable and compostable: the differences

—

It's good to understand the difference in terminology that brands use to describe how their packaging breaks down or can be reused. In a nutshell, 'recyclable' means it can be reused. Certain types of glass and aluminium are endlessly recyclable, whereas most plastics can only be recycled up to a maximum of three times. Bioplastics are generally non-recyclable.

'Biodegradable' means the product breaks down, however it's mainly only under certain conditions and can take anything from a few months to decades. It would be helpful to have more transparent information on brand websites.

'Compostable' is a generalised term meaning that it can decompose at the same rate as a natural material. The problem is that many products labelled 'compostable' can't go in your compost pile in the garden. They have to be sent to an industrial compostable facility, where the conditions are right for that product to decompose properly. More specific labelling is required.

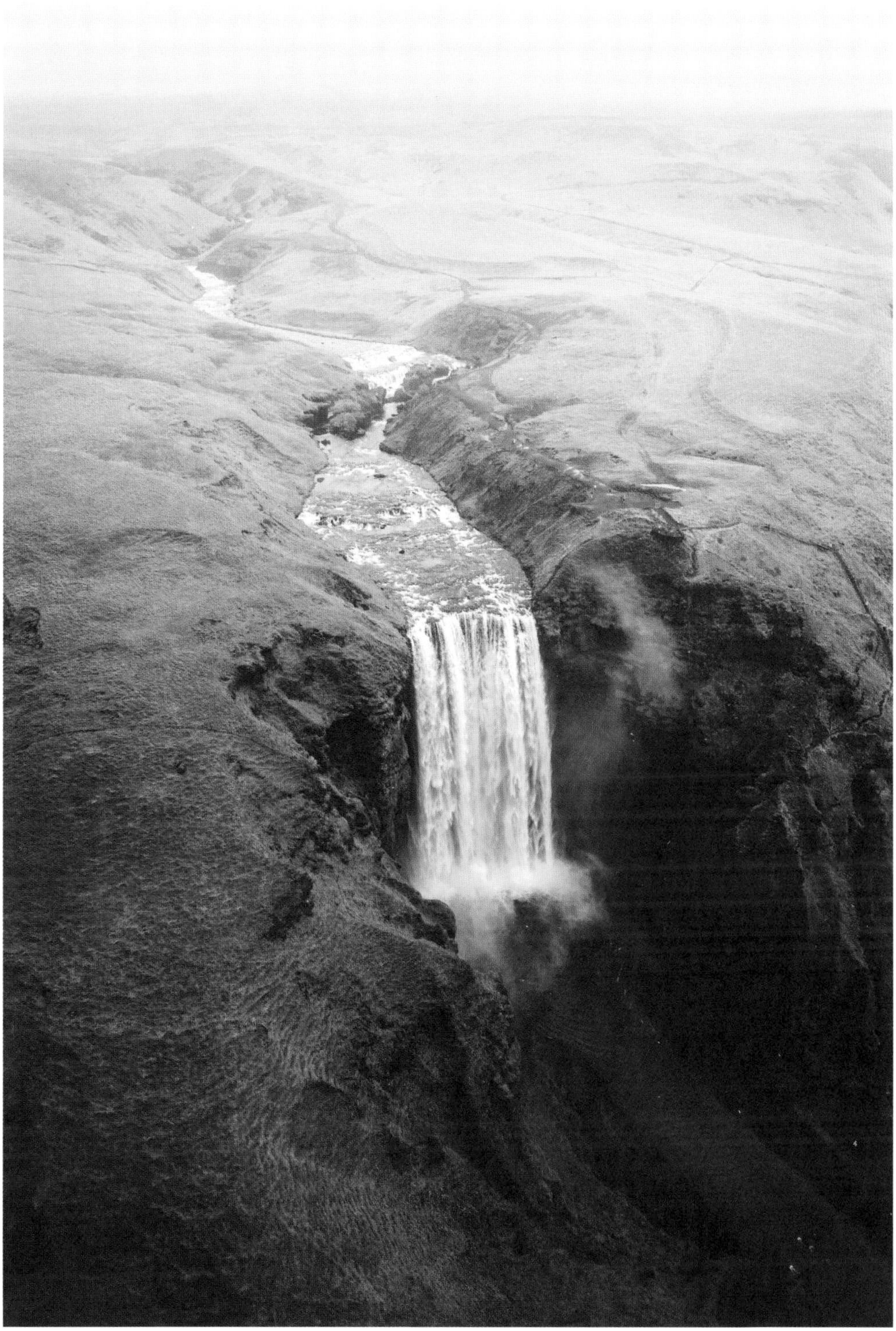

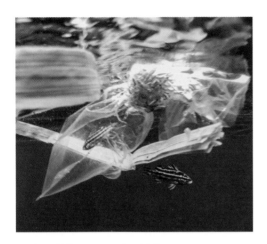

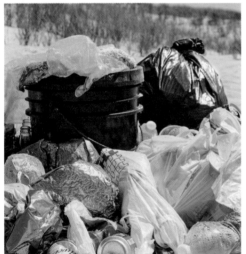

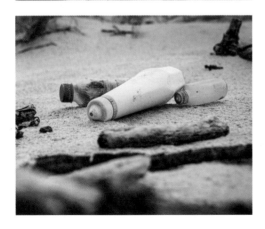

Plastic packaging

All materials have an environmental impact, so it's not just about substituting materials, it's about actually cutting down on what we buy. Let's take a look at the main material that is used in beauty packaging, plastic. Brands house your products in plastic as it's good for stabilising the ingredients inside, it's lightweight so cheaper to post than other materials, and it will arrive on your doorstep without the fear of it being smashed or squashed. So it's great for brands – but not the planet. The process of making plastic requires the use of fossil fuels, which today are being excavated using ways that damage the environment, like fracking. Some plastic beauty packaging can be recycled but it can only be recycled up to three times maximum, and often only once, due to degradation after each use. A lot of brands still use single use (virgin) plastics, which are made primarily from petrochemicals. The other popular option is post-consumer recycled (PCR) plastic, which comes from recycled plastic. Due to the degradation of plastic, often brands will add virgin plastic to the mix of PCR in order to increase the quality of the packaging. They will shout about being 50% PCR and expect a huge round of applause, but it's just not good enough. Spend your hard earned cash on products using 100% PCR packaging or, even better, plastic free or refillable brands.

If plastic packaging is recyclable curbside, it will have a symbol of a triangle of arrows stamped on it with a number inside. This is called the Mobius loop. Use this symbol to check with your council whether you can throw it in your recycling bin. Below is a guide to the most common symbols. Where it indicates 'check', do exactly that with your local home recycling programme so you know whether or not you can place it in your bin. Unfortunately the symbols on beauty packaging are often so small you'll need a magnifying glass. Brands, please don't act like it's an inconvenience; make it bigger, we need to see this stuff!

'Making packaging more recyclable is a step forward, but making more recyclable packaging isn't.' Louise Edge, *Greenpeace*

If the packaging is unmarked or has an empty recycle triangle logo, the only way to find out whether it's recyclable is to ask the brand what material it is made from. You will then need to check with your local authority. Please don't assume this packaging can be recycled curbside or it could contaminate that recycling stream. Manufacturers who buy recycled plastic will pay less for contaminated plastics, or they won't buy them at all. Throw it in the rubbish bin if you can't deliver it to a specialist recycling scheme, but do not chance it in your recycling bin else you'll contaminate the whole load. Try and avoid buying unlabelled plastic in the future.

Specialist recycling

Specialist recycling is a process conducted by various companies who have access to the correct mechanical facilities to reuse hard-to-recycle packaging. For example, TerraCycle are a specialist recycling company that partner with several brands to offer in-store recycling boxes, or you can send your empties directly to them. Other brands encourage customers to post their empties back to them, which they will then recycle. Great as it sounds, my problem with this is that it relies on consumers to put in the extra effort to deliver the beauty packaging to these schemes. Some companies give incentives to return empties by offering discounts or free products, but my experience is that consumers, on the whole, won't do this. Unless brands and local councils make it easy, the majority of people will just bin it. However, as it is our only option at the moment to prevent millions of items of beauty packaging going into landfill, take a deep breath, get online and find your nearest schemes,

then every time you go near a facility, drop them off. Of course, if you cut down your beauty consumption, there won't be as much packaging to contend with in the first place.

Refillable beauty

If you are lucky enough to live near a refillable store, you know how good it feels to save money and be able to reuse your containers time and time again, rather than throwing them into recycling or landfill. Alongside household products, many beauty products like shampoos, conditioners, body washes, bath products and body lotions can be refilled. My local store even offers refills on cleansers and moisturisers. Use an existing container to collect your refillables. Invest in some cool glass jars or beautiful vintage glass bottles. I love old crystal decanters by my bath, full of body washes, soaks, salts and oils. Large amber glass jars or clear jars are simple, stylish

> ### RECYCLING CODES
>
> **PETE 1 (Polyethylene terephthalate)** – widely recycled
>
> **HDPE 2 (High-density polyethylene)** – often recycled
>
> **LDPE 4 (Low-density polyethylene)** – sometimes recycled
>
> **PP 5 (Polypropylene)** – sometimes recycled
>
> **V 3** – non-recycled
>
> **PS 6 (Polystyrene)** – non-recycled
>
> **OTHER 7** – non-recycled policy in place

OUR BEAUTIFUL PLANET

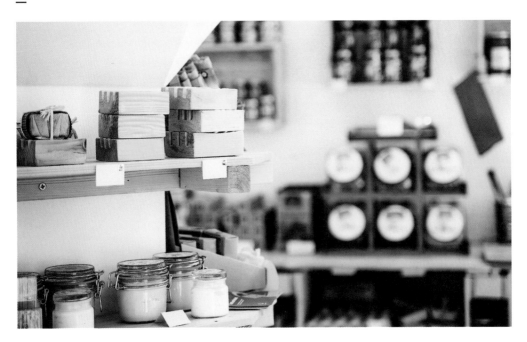

and will look great lined up together. Label your bottle or jar with a brown parcel tag tied around the top with twine – gorgeous! Just make sure you work out how much liquid your bottle holds, as refillable stores sell by liquid measurement.

I'm also seeing refillable stations in hair salons, and some supermarkets are offering this service in partnership with certain brands. Loop is a company set up by the founder of recycling company TerraCycle. Essentially, you buy the product, but rent the packaging. You purchase a moisturiser, for example, which is delivered in a carbon-neutral mode of transport. When your product is nearly used, Loop will deliver another. You return the used bottle to be cleaned and used again.

The beauty industry is also starting to catch on to refillable cosmetics, but we need more brands to get on board. You purchase your product, then when it's finished, instead of throwing the packaging away, you simply replace the contents. This works well for palettes, usually eyeshadows or blushers, where your product comes in an aluminium pan that you place in the palette. When it's finished, you replace the eyeshadow pan, clean out the old aluminium pan and put it in your recycling bin. I'm also seeing more lipstick brands and powder products offering refillables too. Keep researching as more and more brands will follow suit. Juni Cosmetics, for example, has launched a plastic-free lipstick with packaging made from pure aluminium, so once you have used up your lippie, pop it straight into your recycling bin. Zero waste! Shampoo bars are also a great example, where brands have listened to the consumer and created a plastic-free delivery system. Bars are the original way we would have cleaned our hair, so it's nothing new.

Sustainable packaging options

Aluminium
Aluminium is a brilliant, endlessly recyclable material, which doesn't degrade, so is therefore a more sustainable packaging choice for beauty

products. Of course, recycled aluminium is even better, as it requires only 8 per cent of the energy used to make new aluminium. If it does end up in your rubbish bin and incinerated, aluminium metal ash is collected and sent off for recycling. Brilliant! If it ends up in your rubbish bin and in landfill, it takes less time to break down than glass or plastic (over a million years and 500 years respectively). Problems arise when products housed in aluminium have a plastic barrier layer to stabilise the ingredients inside (see below). This turns a perfectly recyclable aluminium tube into a mixed material container, which is non-recyclable curbside.

Glass

Clear, brown, green and blue glass are all easily recycled in your curbside recycling bin. Glass is endlessly recyclable, so choose this option and again you are a sustainable superhero. Remember though to remove any plastic pumps, pipettes and screw caps before you recycle.

Outer and inner packaging

There are plenty of brilliant eco-friendly options out there now, like seed paper, hemp boxes, fibres and compostable chips, so if you receive an item in the post that arrives surrounded by polystyrene chips or foam inserts complain to the company and swap to a more sustainably minded brand.

Packaging is a planetary problem

Microplastics

Microplastics are used by cosmetic manufacturers as cheap fillers and emulsifying agents. When used in wash-off cosmetics, they travel straight from our bathroom drains into our sewer system. Our wastewater treatment plants are not designed to filter them out. Once in our waterways, they are not biodegradable and attract and absorb toxic chemicals. The microplastics get ingested by marine life, and if we consume the marine life, they eventually end up inside our bodies.

Microplastics are also ingested by wildlife, which can result in fatal health issues like intestinal blockages and punctured organs. We do not yet have an understanding of the implications of microplastics to human health, but the United Nations Environment Programme states there is evidence to suggest toxicity in mammals, including humans (see the box below).

Of course brands are not going to advertise the use of microplastics, nor will they make it transparent, as it would deter us from buying them. So how can we avoid products that use microplastics?

Magnets

These are used prolifically in beauty packaging. They weight lipstick bullets to make them feel luxurious, secure refillable eye shadows in a palette and create that superb 'snap' shut mechanism on compacts. More recently, they've been used on false eyelashes that stay together without using glue and as an ingredient in face masks. Magnets cannot be recycled nor can any packing using them. Email brands and tell them you want to see magnets erased from your beauty products, and spend your money on brands who refuse to use magnets in their packaging.

Here are some other examples of microplastics you may find in your beauty products.:

- Acrylates copolymer
- Acrylates crosspolymer
- Butylene
- Carbomer
- Dimethicone
- Polyethylene
- Methacrylate copolymer
- Methacrylate crosspolymer
- Methyl methacrylate copolymer
- Methyl Methacrylate Crosspolymer

Repurposing your packaging

—

To be a sustainable superhero, the best thing you can do over and above recycling, is repurpose. That is, to use the packaging you buy for other long-term uses. You'd be surprised at how your bottles and jars can be incredibly useful around your home. Remove any remaining product (I find a small spatula useful for this), and dispose in your rubbish bin. Never put remaining products down the sink or the toilet as they can contribute to the fatberg problem in our sewers. Ensure the container is clean.

Uses

Pipette bottles – non-recyclable in your home recycling, so keep pipette bottles for homemade tinctures, cooking oil infusions such as truffle or chilli oil, or to make your own facial oil blends.

Glass bottles – remove labels and repurpose as a vase, fill with a homemade bath oil and if the bottle neck is wide enough, it's a great home for bath salts.

Product boxes – make great drawer dividers (à la Marie Kondo) – think lingerie drawers. They can also be repurposed as gift boxes. Outside the home, you can use them to store small change or gloves in your car.

Mascara tubes – once clean, you can make your own lash and brow treatment by filling it with castor oil.

Mascara wands – can be cleaned and sent to your local wildlife centre where they use them to remove fly eggs and mites from animals in their care. They also make very handy jewellery-cleaning and grout-cleaning items.

Plastic tubs and glass jars – these can be used as planters. If they have lids, they can house anything. Use your imagination.

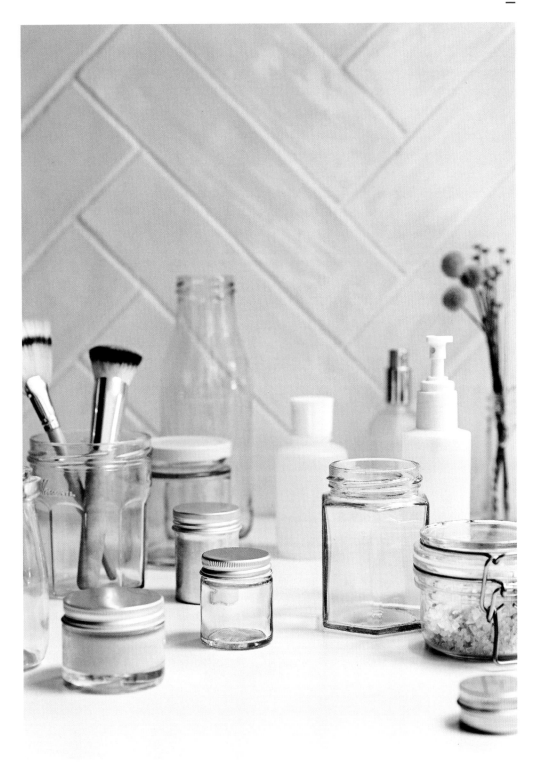

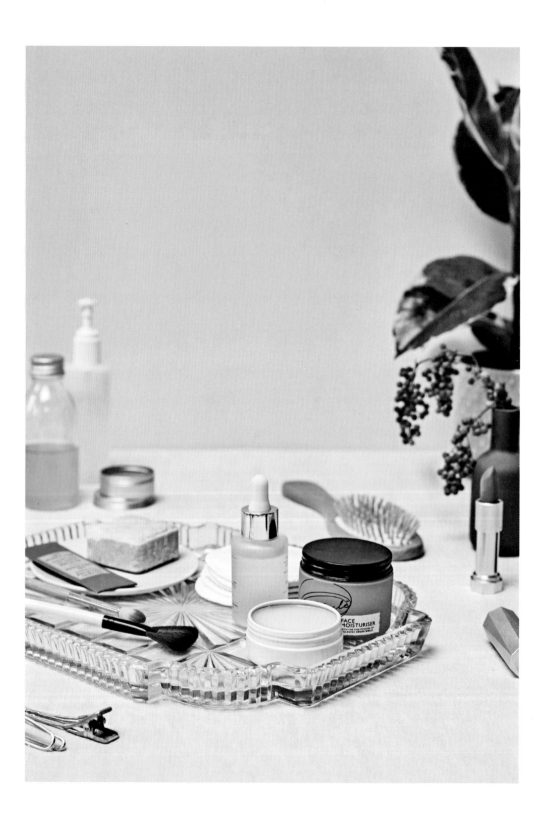

The sustainable self

—

In this part of the book, I'm focusing on sharing my knowledge as a professional make-up artist of 23 years and an ethical artist for the past 10 years. Use this section to learn more about self-care in a sustainable way. Discover what you really need and what you can swap out. I'll coach you through slow beauty make-up techniques, the products you use, skin-care, hair-care and styling. We have looked at ingredients, the environment, packaging and over-consumption in beauty and why we have to reduce. Now we look towards the benefits of having a more edited and mindful routine, and the joy of making your own products. Throughout this section I'll provide recipes for homemade beauty products made from natural ingredients, which will save on packaging, waste, and you'll know exactly what you are putting on your skin. Here you can put your knowledge into practice and be guided on how you can buy less and use better.

Natural and organic

—

I truly believe natural and organic products are kind to us and kind to the planet. However, the terms 'natural' and 'organic' are unregulated in the beauty industry.

A product labelled 'organic' requires a mere 1% of its total ingredients to be organic, and any brand can call itself 'natural'. There is no set criteria for the term 'natural' and without industry standards, the challenge is knowing how natural their product really is.

Formulation school Formula Botanica, describe the different levels of natural. It can be natural ingredients that retain their chemical shape and structure, like cold pressed oils. It can also mean 'naturally derived' ingredients which come from nature, but have undergone a chemical reaction like hydrolysis. Creams and lotions are in this category. Then there is 'nature identical' a synthetic ingredient that is identical in it's chemical structure to that same ingredient found in nature. Salicylic or Sorbic acid can be in this category. The last section are ingredients obtained from plants but processed to mimic a synthetic molecule, for example natural glycols. As a consumer, you have to decide what natural means to you.

Contrary to what some people assume, natural and organic products can be high performance, but are they always the most sustainable option? With deforestation a critical issue, we have to ask ourselves if a synthetic alternative to an ingredient like palm oil would be more sustainable than the natural version. Is a locally produced non-organic product a more sustainable choice than an organic product flown across the world? The beauty industry does not yet have the infrastructure to be wholly sustainable, so ultimately, we as consumers have to choose what our conscience dictates.

When using natural and organic products, I check their provenance and make sure the brand I'm using aligns with my values. Choosing a certified organic brand is a way to protect ourselves from 'greenwashing'; brands promoting a more natural ingredient content and higher ethical values than what really exists. Organic beauty is the formulation of cosmetic products using ingredients grown without the use of Genetically Modified Organisms (GMO), herbicides, synthetic fertilisers and more. The Soil Association set standards for quality of ingredients, organic farming from renewable sources, and human welfare. Organic certifications also come from Cosmos and Nature.

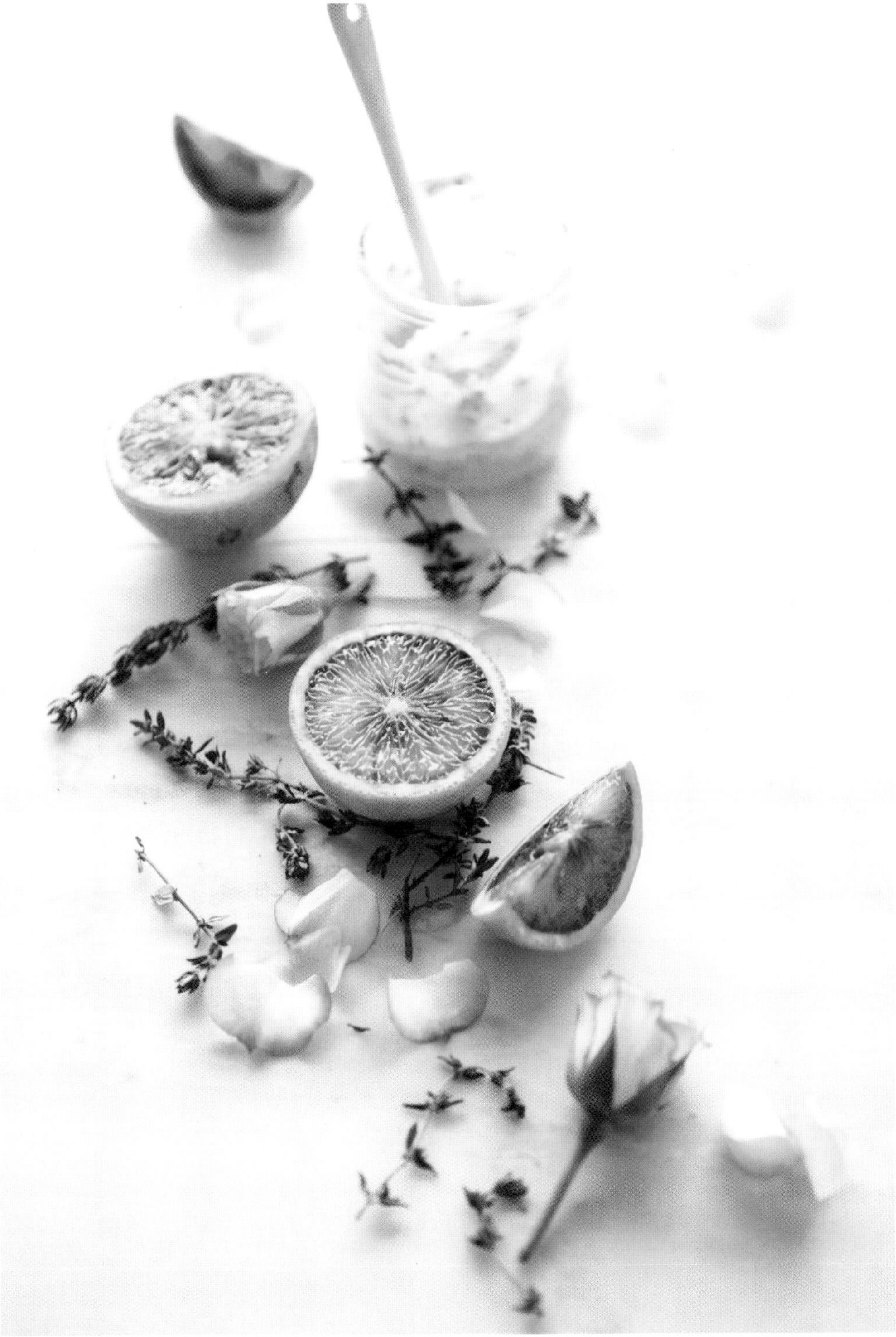

Creating sustainable beauty

—

Homemade beauty products – my story

I admit it. For most of my adulthood, I sneered at the thought of homemade beauty products. I also admit that, as a teenager, I tried making them, but I was soon beckoned by the world of luxurious and expensive products. Besides, why would you smear your face in a concoction of smashed-up bananas and oats, which duly fall off your face like giant flakes of dandruff? I had one misadventure where none of the mix remained on my face. I knew then that my dalliance with homemade masks (or any kitchen beauty product) was over, as I stood surrounded by blobs of what resembled tropical gruel.

Then one day, I had what I like to say was an epiphany, although it's more likely it was a guilt trip. I was cleaning out my bathroom – going through all of the products. Dozens of bottles, jars, tubes… it was endless. Many half-full, dried up, out of date. I was appalled at the waste – my waste. I was confronted with my consumption – and, more importantly, the waste and the negative impact that this gluttony was having on my environment. I had to change. As I questioned what I could do, I recalled my teenage experiments, when I tried to make my own beauty products and bath oils. It got me thinking. It was time to go back into the water and give it another try.

Why make your own beauty products?

Making your own products is a sustainable way of consuming beauty, as you can save on packaging by repurposing. You can eliminate waste by making in small batches which will be completely used, and you'll know exactly what you are putting on your skin because you made it. I've carefully selected these recipes to gradually introduce you to the world of making your own beauty products. If you're anything like me, I just don't have time to faff around in the kitchen conjuring up concoctions with a list of ingredients longer than my legs. I want to pamper myself, but kitchen drudgery is a no-no. So, all of the decadent recipes in this book are simple and quick to create. There are just a couple that require a little extra shopping and commitment, but they deserve inclusion in this section on sheer merit of their efficacy. There are so many benefits to making your own products, but perhaps the main one is that you are creating something for you, and in a world where we often put ourselves last, that is something to celebrate.

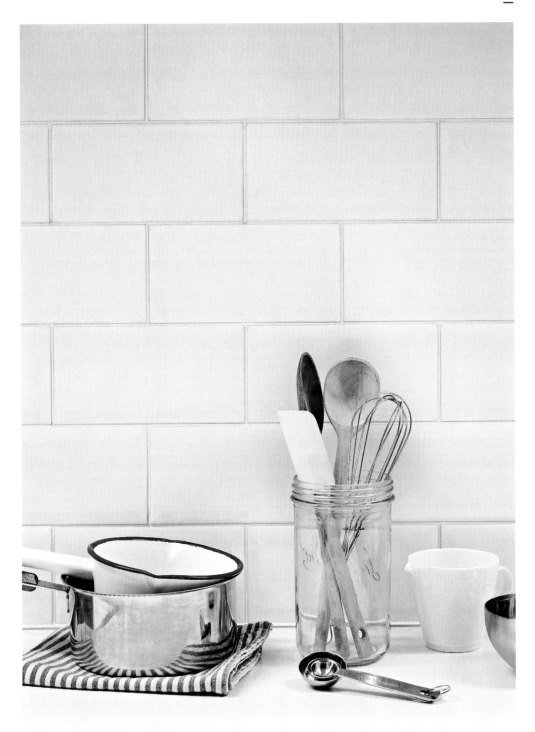

PRACTICAL TIPS

- Store your products out of light and heat.

- Always patch test a new product before slathering it over your skin, especially if you have sensitive skin. Place the product on the inside of your wrist and behind your ear. Wait 24 hours. If at any point your skin becomes sore, itchy, red or blotchy, wet a flannel with cool water and gently remove the product. Keep putting a clean, cool, damp flannel on the area until the redness subsides. Seek medical help if needed. Do not use the product again.

- I've designed these recipes with sensitive skin in mind. If this is your skin type, just eliminate the essential oils. Bacteria forms in water, and water-based products need preservatives, which can be irritating to sensitive skin, so most of these recipes are oil-based. If you have oily skin, don't be afraid of making these recipes.

- Unless the recipe is for dry skin, I've used non-comedogenic oils so they will not clog pores.

- I've made any recipes that don't have to be used immediately waterless. This has kept the recipes very simple; waterless products (anhydrous) have an inbuilt preservation system, which negates the need for a separate preservative. They also last longer!

- Try using clean, sterilised and repurposed jars, spray bottles, pipette bottles and squeezy bottles to store your products.

Sustainability

Creating your own formulations is a sustainable way to consume beauty products. Yes, you have to initially buy the ingredients, but they will go far. You can repurpose other beauty containers like jars and bottles to house your homemade lotions, balms, oils and creams. This will keep them from the recycling process or landfill.

Control

You'll have complete control over your product and can make it totally bespoke to you and your skin needs. All the ingredients will be chosen by you and you'll have complete autonomy over where they come from and what preservative system your product will have.

Budget

You'll save a lot of money by creating your own products and you will have high-quality products at a fraction of the price you would pay in a store. Most of the equipment you will already have in your kitchen; you only need to buy the ingredients you don't have.

Experience

I find making my own products hugely satisfying and fun. It's a wonderful creative outlet for you and your family. People love being given homemade presents. Imagine opening a homemade face balm in a beautiful vintage pot. What's not to love? Follow recipes to start with, then once your confidence builds, you'll feel ready to experiment a little and create your own. I insist that when you're using the fruits of your own labours, you take time to savour and relish the moment. Run baths, light candles, turn the phone off, take a deep breath and simply be.

Bain Marie

Many of the recipes require a bain marie. Also known as a water bath or double boiler, it's a gentle way of heating, melting and emulsifying ingredients together, mostly for cooking but also in beauty recipes too. When choosing the correct glass bowl and saucepan for your bain marie, use a glass bowl that fits snugly on top of the saucepan, but that doesn't come into contact with the water underneath. Place a small amount of water (no less than 1cm/½in depth) into the saucepan, bring to the boil, then reduce the heat so the water is at a gentle simmer. Place the ingredients into the bowl and carefully place it on top of the saucepan. Always use a wooden rather than metal spoon to stir, so that the heat from the bain marie doesn't heat the spoon too.

Melting coconut oil

Boil the kettle and pour hot water carefully into a small bowl until it's a one-third full. Take another smaller bowl and add the desired amount of coconut oil. Place this carefully on top of the bowl of boiling water. Wait a few minutes until the coconut oil has completely melted and is a transparent liquid. Then it's ready to use.

Sterilising jars and bottles for repurposing

Any previous contents should be disposed of in your rubbish bin, not down the sink. Soak the containers in soapy water overnight. If any remnants remain, swish them out with alcohol. You can then sterilise in the oven or by boiling. To boil, the containers must be heatproof, such as glass. Fill a large pot with water, submerge the jars and/or bottles and bring to the boil. Let them boil for 10 minutes before removing them.

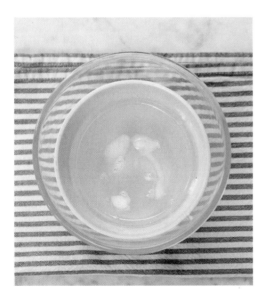

I always let the water cool down naturally, then remove with kitchen tongs. The containers will be very hot, so be careful. Allow to dry completely on clean paper towels before refilling. To oven sterilise, bake the containers for 10–15 minutes at 120°C/250°F. To sterilise plastic containers, dissolve a sterilising tablet in water, then submerge the containers for at least 15 minutes. If you are not using the containers immediately, store them in an airtight sterilised container so they are ready when you need them.

PREPPING YOUR AREA

The step-by-step recipe images in this book were taken with a bit of artistic licence, but if you're making them in your kitchen at home, there are some steps to take so that your products don't become contaminated and you are safe.

- Tie your hair back and cover it with a hairnet.
- Wear a clean apron.
- Protect your eyes with goggles.
- Wear closed shoes.
- Wash your hands.
- Wear single-use disposable nitrile gloves. These, of course, are not very sustainable but necessary for making the beauty products. I would encourage you to seek out your nearest TerraCycle programme for recycling the gloves.
- Wash your utensils and equipment with hot soapy water.
- Clean the floor and counter with dish-washing soap.
- Disinfect your containers, instruments and countertop with alcohol, such as ethanol. Instruments can be steamed by boiling them for 3 minutes if they are heatproof.

THE SUSTAINABLE SELF

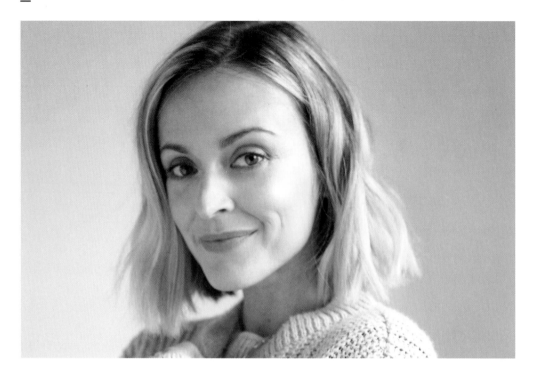

Skincare

—

Skincare is a big subject: the skin is the biggest organ in our body, and there are millions of available products we can choose to put on it. But which products are going to be the best for you to invest in? And how do you know they will work for you and your particular type of skin? A daily healthy skin regime doesn't have to be time consuming, and you don't have to spend a fortune.

Skincare is a great way to connect and check in with yourself. When I'm doing someone's make-up, the first thing I'll do is put my hands on their skin, just for a moment. It gives me an opportunity to tune in. During those seconds, I can sense and feel what their skin needs. I'm all about natural-looking skin – there are no heavy, cakey foundations in my kit – so nourishing my client's skin and encouraging it to look its best is the basis of my personal make-up technique. Having a 'conversation' with your skin is important. Put your clean, dry hands on your face and get to know your skin. In return, it'll let you know what it really needs.

Cleansing

One of the easiest ways to keep your skin looking healthy and radiant is cleansing. Everyone needs to cleanse their skin. Even if you don't wear make-up, your skin needs to be washed of the dirt and bacteria that has accumulated from everyday living. If you don't, it can become clogged and you'll have to deal with break-outs, blackheads, dryness and more. A couple of minutes cleansing has such huge benefits to your skin health. If you wear a lot of make-up, a double cleanse is something to try. The first cleanse removes make-up, and the second cleanse has a deeper cleaning and radiance-boosting action. Yes, you are using more product, but if you get your skin looking it's best, you won't need to wear as much make-up, so view it as a trade-off.

What works best?
The majority of cleansers come in the form of oils, balms, gels, waters, creams and milks. Personally, I prefer oils and balms, especially for dryer skins. Even if you have oily or combination skin, don't dismiss an oil cleanser. Here's why.

Your skin has a thin protective layer called the 'acid mantle' that's made up of amino and lactic acids which mix easily with fatty acids (oils) from the sebaceous glands. These glands secrete oil that protects your skin. The pH level of your skin's acid mantle is around 5.5, which is slightly acidic. When you wash your face with harsh cleansers, which are alkaline, you wash away the oil that protects your skin. You dry it out and it becomes vulnerable to skin issues. Oil has no pH level, so oil-based cleaners will remove dirt without affecting the acid mantle and PH level of your skin. The majority of oils and balms can be used around the eyes (check the packaging), therefore you are investing in a sustainable swap by eliminating a separate eye make-up remover. Soft to use, these are super effective and won't drag the delicate skin around the eyes. If you find using the one product for all irritates the eye, add a separate eye make-up remover to your routine.

Not all oils are created equally, and I'd suggest you go for pure organic, plant-based oils. Never use mineral oils, and even some natural oils, such as grapeseed, can go rancid quickly or others, like argan oil, can contain impurities that disrupt skin. When I can, I always choose jojoba oil. Use a pure organic oil and your skin will feel nourished and cleansed. After using some cleansing products, your skin can feel dry, uncomfortable and tight. You'll never get that with the right oil.

TECHNIQUE: Rub three pumps (or eight drops) of product between your fingertips and onto the skin using sweeping and circular motions. Try to keep the strokes going upwards – don't drag the skin downwards. Lightly sweep your fingers over your closed eyes and don't rub them – gently does it. Personally, I dislike waterproof mascaras, as they are difficult to remove. Avoid them unless you are getting married and suspect you might cry, or if you just can't wear any other mascara. If you do need to remove this stuff, then stick to gently rubbing your lashes only. You do not need to rub your whole eye area to remove mascara. Your first cleanse should remove your make-up, so get in the brows and the sides of the nose.

It's pretty much the same technique for a second cleanse, but here you can concentrate on some facial massage to get the blood flowing to your skin. If you are using botanicals, take some deep breaths and inhale their heavenly aroma. Don't be afraid to use your whole hands. As long as you are not dragging your skin, do what feels good. Remove with a damp flannel. If you already own flannels, use what you have but if you need to purchase new ones, look for hemp face cloths, as much less water is used to produce it than cotton, and it doesn't release microplastics into the waterways like microfibres. I also like using muslin cloths: when past their best, you can repurpose in my healing oat soak recipe (see page 76).

Jojoba facial cleansing oil

Oils are an effective and gentle way to cleanse the skin without leaving that tight, dry feeling you get after using certain cream, gel or foam cleansers. Jojoba oil has a myriad of healing properties, so it is perfect for soothing skin conditions like acne, eczema and psoriasis. The recipe also includes castor oil which contains essential fatty acids that nourish and moisturise, and vitamin E oil is full of anti-oxidants which help reduce scarring and pigmentation. If you want to use this formulation around the eyes, then leave out the essential oils.

Ingredients
– 25ml (1 tbsp plus 2 tsp) jojoba oil
– 40ml (2 tbsp plus 2 tsp) castor oil
– 1 tsp vitamin E oil
– 10 drops essential oil (chamomile, sandalwood, geranium, rose [normal–dry skin], tea tree, lavender, lemon, cypress, juniper [oily skin], optional)

Equipment
– Small jug
– Metal spoon
– Funnel (optional)
– 100ml (3½fl oz) repurposed glass bottle with pump dispenser, sterilised

Method
1. One at a time, pour the jojoba, castor and vitamin E oils into the jug.

2. Mix in the essential oils, if using, and stir with the metal spoon.

3. Pour the liquid into the glass bottle and seal it. You can use a funnel to reduce any spillage, if necessary. Store in a cool dark place for up to 1 year.

4. To use, dispense three pumps of the cleansing oil, or 8 drops, onto your hands and rub them together. Place your hands over your face and massage the oil into your skin in a circular motion to cleanse and remove make-up.

Place a muslin cloth or flannel under warm water and squeeze until the excess water is removed and the cloth is damp, but not wet. Gently remove the cleansing oil from your skin by wiping the cloth across your face until the make-up is removed.

Repeat, if necessary, for stubborn/waterproof make-up.

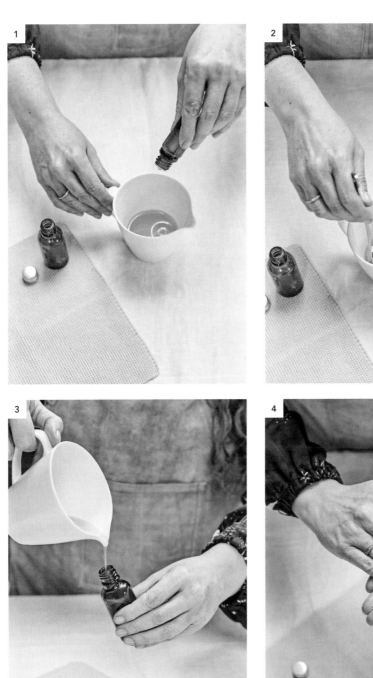

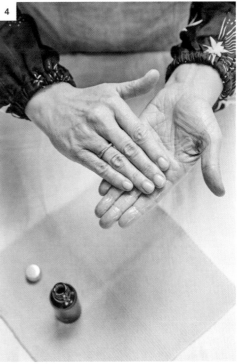

Wipe out wipes!

I despair at the use of disposable wipes – I call it my 'wipe gripe'. Often made of single-use plastics, like polyester, and housed in non-recyclable packaging, disposable wipes are a sustainable no-no. They do not cleanse the skin properly. Just use your regular flannel/cloth and a cleanser. Many single-use cleansing wipes, cleaning wipes, toilet wipes, baby wipes, bum wipes and vag wipes are just flushed down the loo. No! Water UK announced that wipes account for a staggering 93 per cent of the material blocking UK sewers, most of which were built in the Victorian era before we even had toilet paper. Our loos are not bins; they are not designed for wipes. What goes down the loo does not just magically disappear. It goes into our sewers, our rivers, our seas; it becomes microplastics. It's then eaten by plankton, then by fish and then by us. We are ingesting this stuff!

Micellar waters

These are a mixture of soft water and micelles (tiny balls of oil), designed to be used as a cleanser when there is no water available. They're not as efficient as cream, balm, gel or oil cleansers, and not cleansing your skin sufficiently will result in dull clogged skin. Great in a make up artists kit for a quick make up change, but at home, there is no need for them. If you simply can't do without them, just use them to remove make-up, not to cleanse your skin.

Facial cleansing brushes

These rotating brushes are marketed as cleansing devices, but they are actually more like exfoliators. If you use one, treat it like a once- or twice-a-week exfoliator and not a daily cleansing tool. If you over-exfoliate, you risk damaging your skin's protective barrier.

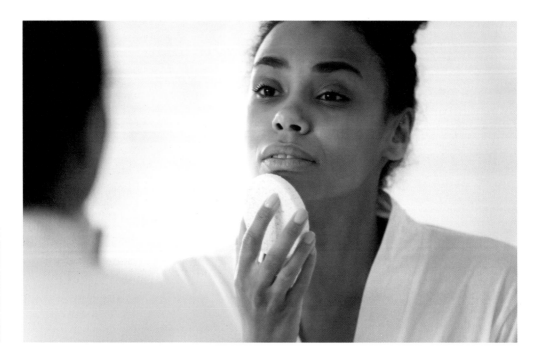

Toning

Toning used to be something that many people either never understood or saw as an unnecessary skincare step. However, these days a good liquid toner is more aligned to the pH of your skin (slightly acidic), and when applied after cleansing, it is supportive in maintaining the skin's balance. Toners containing a lot of alcohol should be avoided, however a little organic alcohol is fine, as are vegetable alcohols such as stearyl, behenyl and cetearyl alcohols, which can brighten the skin. When I say a little, I mean a little! They should never be high up on the INCI list. Avoid SD (specially denatured) alcohol, denatured alcohol, benzyl alcohol and isopropyl alcohol. When choosing a toner for oily skin with naturally derived ingredients, look for gentle astringents instead, such as rose water, mint, apple cider vinegar, witch hazel, tea tree, rose oil and naturally derived salicylic acid. For dryer skins and mature skins I'd recommend hyaluronic acid, aloe, vegetable glycerine and algae. Those with sensitive skin will respond best to calming ingredients, such as aloe, chamomile, cucumber and rose water. Pure rose water is often sold as a toner. If you use this product, please make sure it is of very high quality and not one filled with artificial fragrance. A good natural toner will include antioxidants, ceramides and essential fatty acids.

TECHNIQUE: Toner should be applied to clean skin, so always cleanse first. If your toner has a thicker consistency, you can pour a little bit onto your fingertips and then apply it to your skin in a gentle pressing motion. If your toner is a thinner liquid, apply with a reusable pad sweeping across your skin in upwards movements. Toner is designed to be left on the skin, so don't wash it off. Use it twice a day, morning and evening, on clean skin.

Liquid exfoliators/acid toners

Acid toners, also known as liquid exfoliators, go deeper than regular toners to remove dirt and dead skin cells. If you are happy using an acid toner, they are a sustainable win as they do the job of a 2-in-1 toner and exfoliator, eliminating the need for a separate exfoliating product. A word of caution here. As with any exfoliating product, too much exfoliation is damaging. Start very slowly and, unless specified by a skincare professional, build up to a maximum three times a week, in the evening. If you are happy using daily and your skin is healthy, then who am I to judge, but I personally would suggest less is more. If using acid toners, avoid other exfoliating products such as acid serums, cleansing brushes and facial scrubs. Fast-acting and easy to use, acid toners give quick visible results. However, while pores may look tighter and make-up application is smoother, this could be due to moisture loss. They are usually water-based, so they evaporate quickly and don't provide long-lasting benefits. This loss of water can leave your skin feeling tight and dehydrated. If you want to use an acid exfoliator, consider substituting with an acid serum, which is less hard-hitting and longer lasting. Not just for the face, acid toners are a good treatment for keratosis pilaris (bumps on the skin often referred to as 'chicken skin'), caused by dead skin cells plugging hair follicles.

The term 'acid' here refers to alpha hydroxy acids (AHAs), like glycolic acid or lactic acid, and/or beta hydroxy acids (BHAs), such as salicylic acid, which deeply cleanses the pores, ridding your skin of dead skin cells and excess oil production. These acids contain many beneficial ingredients like exfoliants and anti-inflammatory agents, which create brighter, fresher radiant skin. Acid toners are powerful products and, used wisely, can be hugely beneficial. Always purchase from reputable brands and do not make your own. The acids that will work best for you will depend on your skin type: salicylic (from willow bark) if you

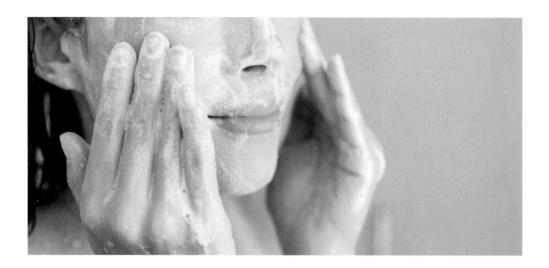

Facial scrubs

have acne-prone skin; lactic acid for sun damage and fine lines; and glycolic and lactic acid if you have sensitive skin. Poly hydroxy acids (PHAs) are much more gentle, so suitable if you have really sensitive skin. Please note that in its natural form, lactic acid is derived from milk and so it's not a vegan ingredient. Most lactic acids used in skincare now are synthetic, so are vegan.

Designed to be used once or twice a week, these products slough off dead skin cells and encourage new cell growth. Many people think of them as an outdated method of exfoliation, which has been replaced with acid toners and serums. However, for those that are not comfortable using acid products, scrubs are a great option. Regular use gives clearer skin, fewer visible lines and wrinkles and enhances the performance of other skincare products. The application of make-up is also smoother.

TECHNIQUE: Take a reusable pad and pour on enough toner to make it wet, but not sopping or dripping. Sweep across your skin in upward movements. You will feel a tingling sensation, but if that turns to stinging, rinse off the product immediately and discontinue use. Remember to avoid other exfoliating products such as acid serums or retinol treatments, but if you are using them, be careful of exposure to sunlight. Consider using an acid serum instead of a liquid acid toner, as the level of humectants (a substance used to keep things moist) in the serum will hydrate the new cells while exfoliating the old ones.

TECHNIQUE: After cleansing, keep the skin damp or spray with a facial spritz. Take a small amount of scrub and massage in circular motions over the face and neck. Wash off with a damp cloth or flannel.

Facial mists/spritzes

I absolutely love a facial spritz: the fine mist on the skin traps in moisture, helping the skin to feel hydrated. Use after cleansing but before applying a serum. Applying a cool spritz first thing in the morning is a great wake-up treatment (especially if you've kept yours in the fridge). You can also pop it on between layers of products. I almost always use spritzes on clients' skin before applying a moisturiser. It helps to plump and hydrate, and that makes for a better make-up application. Most spray bottles operate with a non-recyclable pump, which will need to be disposed of correctly. Consider making your own using repurposed packaging.

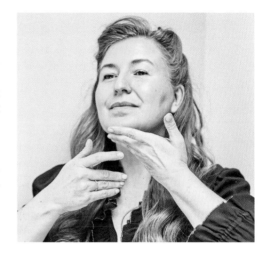

Serums

Think of serums like super-charged skincare. The active ingredients work hard for your skin and the consistency allows deeper penetration and better results. Serums come in the form of oils, gels and lotions, often in a pump or pipette bottle.

> **TECHNIQUE:** Use one or two pumps. Spread the serum between your fingertips then sweep all over your face and neck. Apply after cleansing and toning, but before moisturising.

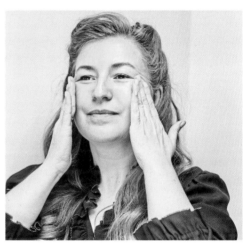

Acid serums

Acid serums are exfoliating serums used to deep clean pores and encourage cell renewal, promoting clearer, brighter skin. They are a good sustainable swap, as they negate the need for a separate exfoliating product or toner. A little tingling is normal when you first use them, but if this continues or becomes a stinging sensation, then scale back their use or stop using them altogether. Signs of overuse are simultaneous redness and dryness.

TECHNIQUE: Use acid serums after cleansing and at night, as this is the time for skin repair. AHA acids can make the skin more sensitive to the sun's rays, so if you use any acid products in the summer, make sure you protect your skin with sunscreen. Place an edamame-sized amount on your fingertips, smooth between your fingers and sweep over the skin. Pay special attention to the sides of the nose where product can gather. Avoid the eyes unless the product can be used in that area. Follow up with a moisturiser.

A skin elixir for all ages

I dislike the term 'anti-ageing'. It only serves to fuel our society's desire for youth, which takes away the enjoyment and appreciation of the wisdom of our years. I much prefer the term 'pro-ageing'; it sounds so much more positive. This serum is a gorgeous elixir for skin of all ages. I've kept it oil-based to eliminate the need for preservatives.

Ingredients
- 4 tsp rosehip oil
- 1 tsp argan oil
- 1 tsp vitamin E oil
- 2 tsp buriti oil
- 1 tsp CBD oil
- 1 tsp borage oil
- 5 drops essential oil of your choice (optional)

Equipment
- Small glass jug
- Metal spoon
- Funnel
- 50ml/1¾fl oz repurposed glass bottle with pipette, sterilised

Method
1. One at a time, add the rosehip, argan, vitamin E, buriti, CBD and borage oils to the glass jug and stir together with the metal spoon.

2. Add the essentials oils, if using, and mix well.

3. Using a funnel, pour the mixture into the glass bottle and store in a cool dark place.

To use, place a few drops of the serum onto your fingers and rub together. Rub into your face and leave the oils to absorb into your skin. It can be used anywhere on the face and body.
.

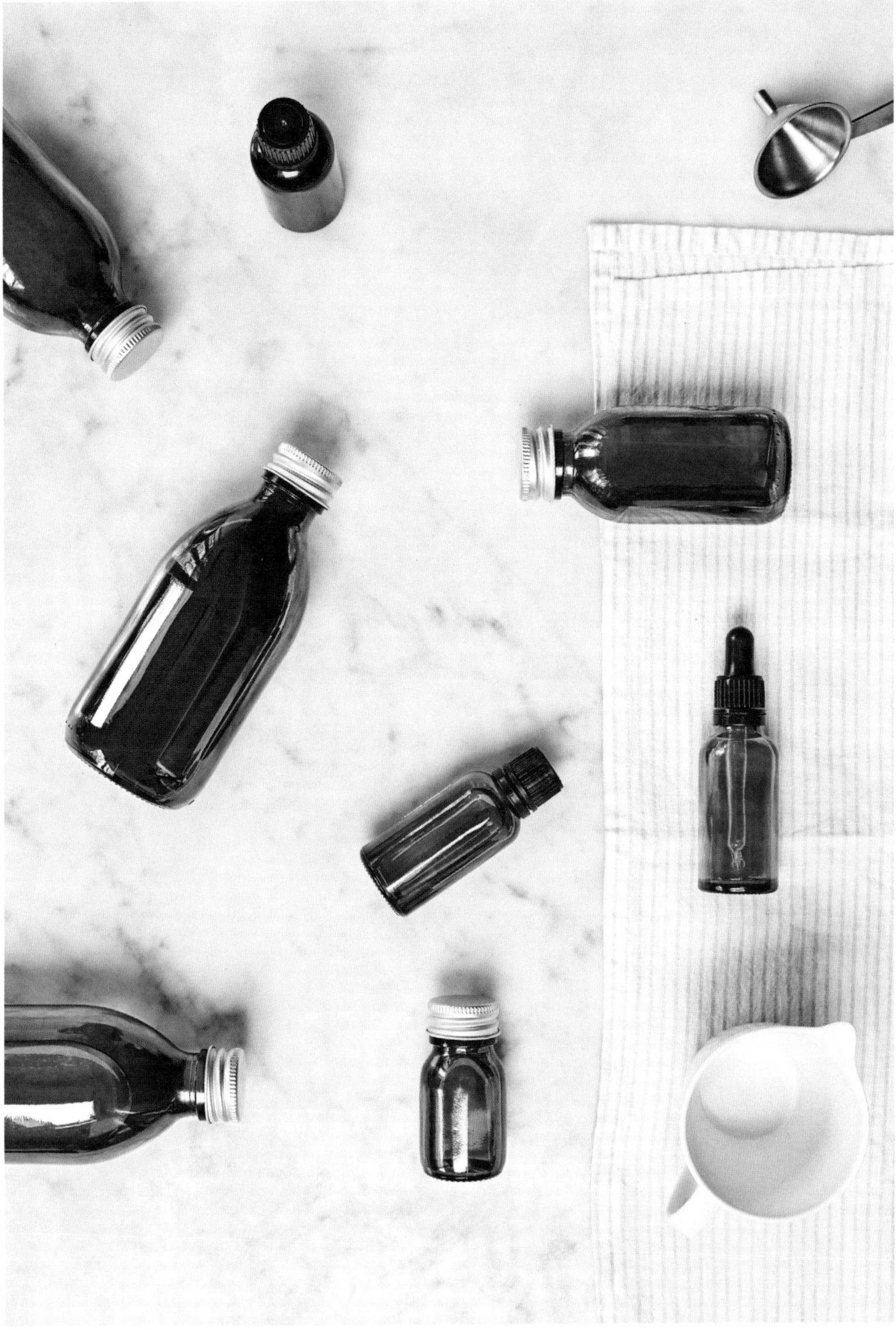

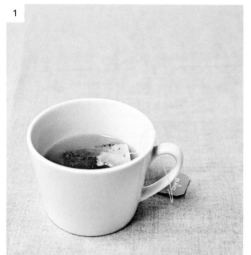

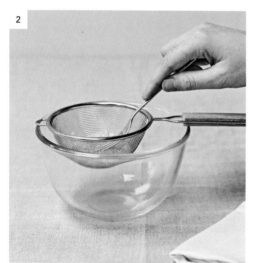

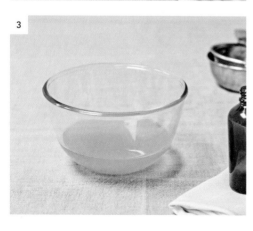

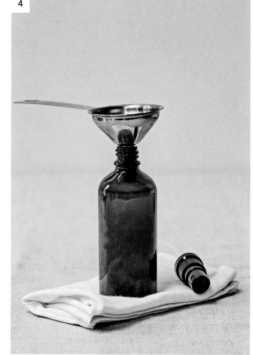

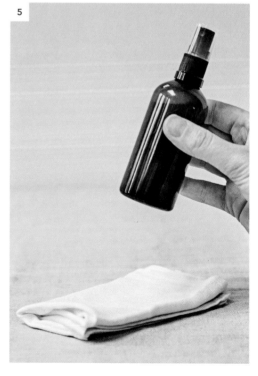

A refreshing all-season spritz of rosewater, cucumber & green tea

A fine mist of this fresh, zingy yet moisturising rosewater, cucumber and green tea blend is amazing for cooling the face on hot summer days, moisturising winter-dry skin, ameliorating the effects of air conditioning and also soothing and calming the skin during a menopausal flush. As well as all this, I love to use the spritz as a toner, and under moisturiser as it's more effective to moisturise over wet skin. The combined active properties of the ingredients in this recipe are plentiful and all-purpose. The spritz soothes, calms and hydrates the skin, as well as balancing the pH level. All this, and it's packed with antioxidants. I hope you enjoy this dreamy all- season mist as much as I do.

Note: As a test, spritz your wrists first and see if your skin reacts after 24 hours. There are three ingredients listed below (witch hazel, lemon juice and peppermint essential oil), which can be eliminated from the recipe for those with very sensitive skin.

Ingredients
– 1 green tea bag
– ¼ cucumber, peeled and cubed
– 120ml (4fl oz/½ cup) rose water
– 1 tsp witch hazel (optional)
– ½ tsp lemon juice (optional)
– 2 drops peppermint essential oil (optional)

Equipment
– Cup or mug
– Masticating juicer (optional)
– Small saucepan
– Fork
– Muslin (cheesecloth) or fine sieve
– Mixing bowl
– Funnel
– Spray atomiser bottle, sterilised

Method

1. Place the tea bag in the cup and pour over 120ml (4fl oz/ ½ cup) boiling water. Set aside to cool.

2. Pass the cucumber through a masticating juicer (if using). Alternatively, cook the peeled and cubed cucumber in the saucepan over a low heat, to soften. Using a fork, strain the mixture through the muslin or sieve into a bowl. For really smooth results strain a second time .

3. Mix in the rose water and cool green tea. Add the witch hazel, lemon juice and peppermint oil, if using.

4. Using a funnel, carefully pour the liquid into the bottle and screw on the atomiser.

5. Shake vigorously. Store in the fridge and use within 3 weeks. If, within this time you notice a change in scent, texture or appearance, it's time to make a new batch.

To use, hold the bottle about 10cm (4in) away from the face and spray liberally, keeping your eyes and lips closed. Bend your elbow up to a 90-degree angle for the right distance from your face. Close your eyes and mist all over your face. If you are applying another skin care product on top, do this while your skin is still a little damp to lock in the moisture.

A 'night-scented' face serum for all skin types

This gorgeous and dreamy-scented skin soak features aloe vera mixed with almond oil, which will help to keep your skin supple, soft and deeply hydrated. It will also firm the skin and diminish lines. The exotic aroma of ylang ylang with the fresh twist of lavender oil is evocative and lulls you into dreamland while feeding the skin. Use on your face and over neck areas, décollatage and your boobs. Omit the essential oils, if you want to use around the eyes or if you have sensitive skin.

Note: You can make a larger batch to use all over the body.

Makes 50ml (1¾fl oz)

Ingredients
– 1 tbsp aloe vera 10:1
  concentrate
– 3 tbsp fractionated
  coconut oil
– 2 tbsp sweet almond oil
– 1 tsp vitamin E oil
– 3 drops ylang ylang
  essential oil
– 1 drop lavender
  essential oil

Equipment
– Mixing bowl
– Hand whisk
– 50ml (1¾fl oz)
  repurposed pump
  bottle or jar, sterilised

Method
1–2. Put the aloe vera concentrate and the oils in the mixing bowl.

3–4. Whisk for 30 seconds. Using the funnel, decant into the pump bottle or jar.

To use, massage a small amount into selected area of skin.

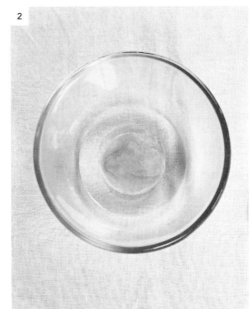

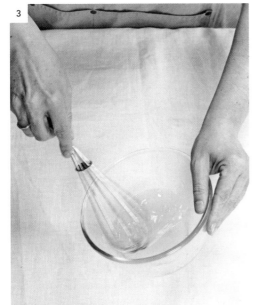

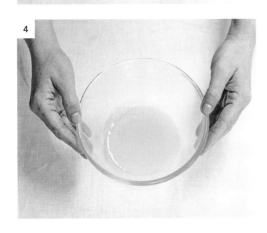

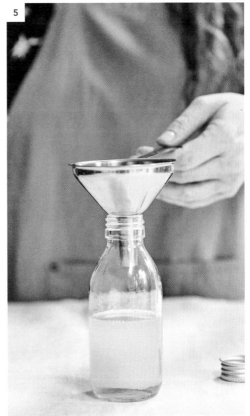

Facial oils

A great facial oil is pure heaven. I love mine to include quality essential oils, but if you have highly sensitive skin or an allergy to an essential oil, then stick to one without. Don't think that essential oils will make a facial oil even oilier. A high-quality essential oil will have a molecular structure that is more like a gas, which is easily absorbed; therefore, it won't sit on top of your skin. Why I love a good-quality organic facial oil is that you can tell your skin loves it. It improves the look and feel of skin in seconds. This is also a great time to do some facial massage with your fingertips or a gua sha tool. If you have oily skin, don't dismiss facial oils; your skin needs them. A good one will improve the over-production of oil – think of it as like cancelling out like. If you don't enjoy the feel of it, add a couple of drops into your moisturiser, or only apply it at night.

TECHNIQUE: Place two to three drops of oil on your fingertips, press and move lightly between your fingertips and fingers to disperse, then press quite firmly all over the skin. Don't drag your fingers. If your product contains essential oils, make the most of that exquisite aroma and take a few deep breaths in through the nose and out through the mouth as you are applying. If you are including moisturiser in your routine, and I suggest you do, your oil product should go on first.

Eye creams

The thinner skin around the eye shows one of the first signs of ageing. Most of us over the age of 25 will benefit from using a product around the eye area. Lifestyle and genetics will dictate whether you will have dark circles, puffiness, wrinkles – or possibly all three. A good product can help, but nothing can override genetics I'm afraid. If you don't really have any of these issues, then make a sustainable swap and skip a separate eye product. Use your facial serum and moisturiser around your eyes instead (as long as it's safe to use – check the instructions). If using a separate product, I prefer a thinner consistency for the eye area, so I like an eye serum or gel. Creams and lotions are also available, so it depends on what you find most comfortable to use.

TECHNIQUE: Use a very small amount, like half a grain of rice. Squeeze it on to your ring finger and press against your other ring finger. Then lightly apply all around your orbital bone, starting from nearest the nose and working outwards. Don't be tempted to place the product closer to the eyeball area as you could risk irritating your eye. The ring finger is advised for application, as it's the finger with the least amount of pressure when applying products to delicate areas. Apply after cleansing and toning and before moisturiser, but it is up to you whether you apply before or after a serum.

Eye patches

These serum-infused patches are designed to hydrate and treat fine lines. They can be packaged in plastic and the patches themselves are non-recyclable, so a better option is to choose those packaged in a recyclable tub. The patches themselves will have to be thrown away, but the tub can be recycled. Organic cotton patches are another more sustainable option as they are reusable, however consider the water and energy used to make the cotton. Silicone patches can be reused; however, once the silicone has been used to its capacity, it will need to be sent off for specialist recycling. A better idea is to simply place a thicker amount of serum under the eye area and remove the excess after ten minutes.

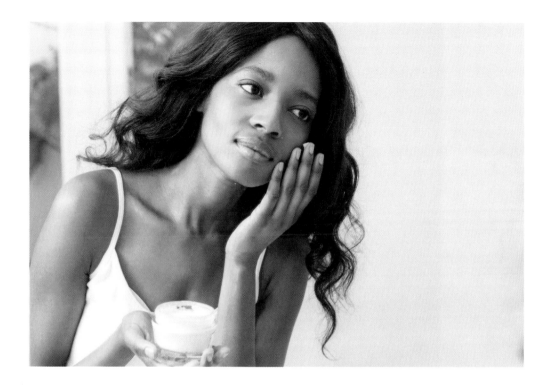

Moisturisers

Whatever our skin type, we all need a moisturiser to comfort and protect the skin. Oil and moisture are two different things, so you can have oily skin that is also dehydrated. Do you need a separate day and night moisturiser? Not really. Night creams are usually heavier than day creams, so instead of a separate night cream, I would suggest a sustainable swap by using a serum then your facial oil at night, as they both have greater skin benefits. If you do want to moisturise at night, then you can just use your day moisturiser over your serum or oil.

Similarly, your moisturiser and serum can be used on your neck and décolletage; you won't need a separate product.

TECHNIQUE: Consider a pot rather than a pump dispenser for your moisteriser as you are more likely to be able to recycle the packaging kerbside. Using clean hands, take an edamame-sized amount, spread between your fingertips and fingers to disperse the product, then press into the skin and neck and sweep over the skin in upwards movements. Use after cleanser, toner, serum and/or oil.

THE SUSTAINABLE SELF

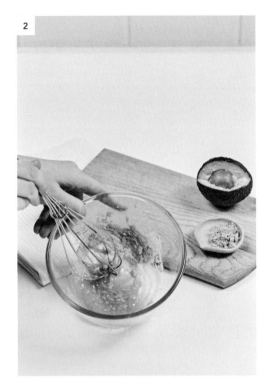

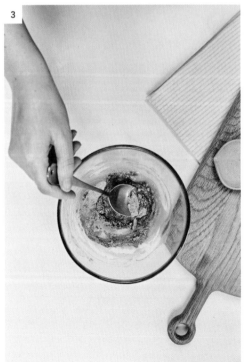

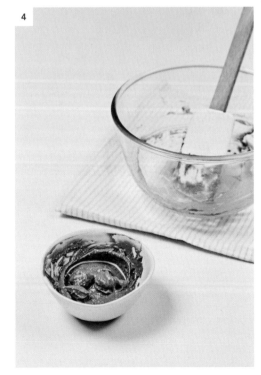

Double 'A' face paste

It doesn't get simpler than my double 'A' face paste, a luxurious and restorative face mask with only three ingredients: avocado, agave nectar and green clay.

Avocados contain an abundance of powerful ingredients. When used in a mask, they work to deep clean and moisturise, while their vitamins E and C repair and protect the skin against UV damage. They also stimulate collagen production, minimising the appearance of fine lines and rejuvenating and conditioning the skin.

The agave nectar contains glycolic acid and antioxidants. It absorbs into the skin quickly and leaves it looking fresh and younger, and also eliminates any excess oil. Additionally, agave works on controlling acne and reduces inflammation of the skin. What more could you ask from these two super-skin power players?

The green clay gently exfoliates and cleanses the pores, restoring balance to the skin. This clay is great for combination skin, but gentle enough for all skin types.

Makes 1 mask

Ingredients
– ¼ avocado (fully ripe and soft)
– 1 tbsp agave nectar
– 1 tsp green clay

Equipment
– Mixing bowl
– Fork
– Hand whisk (or blender)
– Spatula
– Repurposed glass jar, bowl or jam jar with lid

Method
1. Place the avocado quarter in the bowl and mash until smooth with a fork (you can eat the rest or make a larger quantity of mask to use on the hair and body).

2. Add the agave nectar and whisk together well until a smooth paste develops. Alternatively, you can use a blender.

3. Add the green clay and mix together to form a paste.

4. Immediately decant into the glass jar, scraping out all the contents of the bowl with a spatula to make sure you do not waste any. Seal the jar with the lid to avoid discoloration. This paste is best used on the day you make it.

To use, spread the paste generously over the face. Leave to absorb into the skin for 10–15 minutes.

Remove the mask with a warm, damp flannel or face cloth and rinse your face with cold water.

Tip: As your avocados need to be ripe and soft for this, it's a good way to use up avocados that are on the way out!

A nourishing oat face mask

When you're making a batch of my healing oat soak for sensitive skin (see page 76), try to keep some oat powder back for this recipe. Oats are an effective alternative to soaps and detergents, so are great for nourishing tired skin and wonderful in a face mask like this one. Oats contain antioxidants and anti-inflammatory compounds.

Makes 1 mask

Ingredients
– 2 tsp ultra-fine organic ground oats or oat powder
– 2 tsp castor oil

Equipment
– Food processor
– Mixing bowl
– Meta spoon
– Face cloth

Method
1. Place the ground oats in the bowl. Add the castor oil and mix until it becomes a paste.

2. Apply to your clean, dry face using your fingertips, avoiding your eyes and lips. Leave for 10 minutes.

3. Wipe off with a damp face cloth or rinse off with cold water. Pat dry.

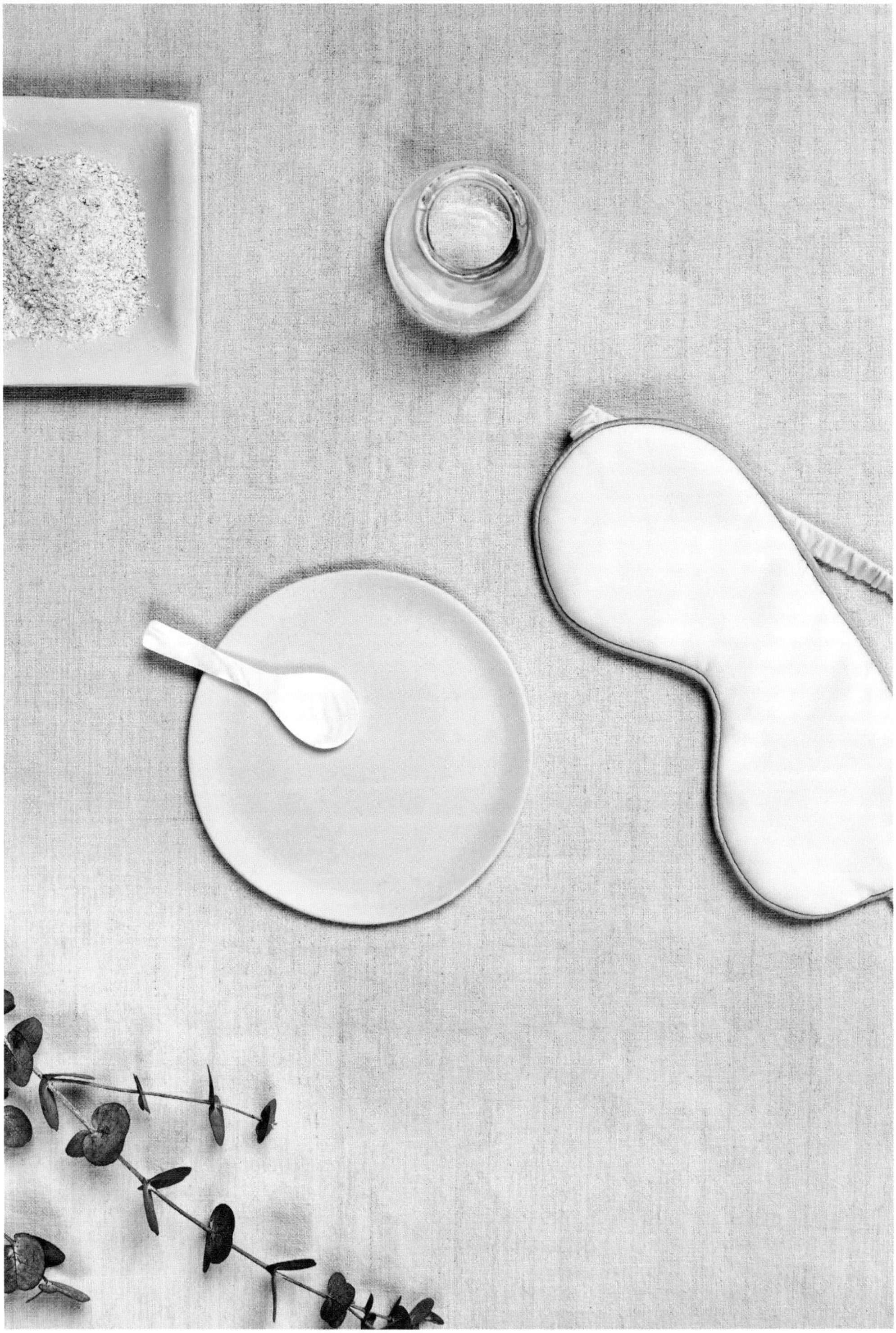

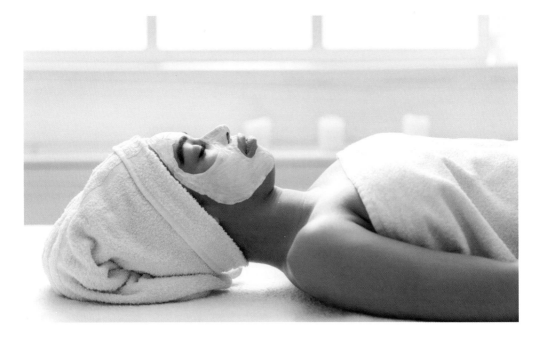

Facial masks and sheet masks

Designed to be used a couple of times a week, facial masks can give your skin an extra boost. However, if you are really looking after your skin, you shouldn't need to purchase one and can alternatively make your own.

Sheet masks are thin sheets coated in serum, with holes for eyes, nose and mouth. They are designed for single use which makes them a sustainable no-no. Sheet masks rarely have recyclable packaging and the mask itself will have to be thrown away.

Spot treatments

Some brand spot treatments are effective, but none in my opinion work as well as tea tree oil. This useful antibacterial and antiseptic natural essential oil is one to keep in your beauty larder as it's very multitasking. You can treat breakouts, cuts, use it in hair rinses and mouth rinses, and even clean your worktops with it, so swap out all spot treatments in favour of sustainable tea tree oil from a reputable brand. Always dilute it in a carrier oil before placing on the skin, hair or scalp as it's a strong oil and too potent for direct use. If you've never used tea tree oil before, please do a patch test beforehand. If you have very sensitive skin, then proceed with caution.

YOUR ESSENTIAL SKIN-CARE LIST:

– Cleanser
– Toner and exfoliator, or acid toner or serum (you only need either one)
– Facial spritz (you don't need this with a toner)
– Serum
– Facial oil
– Moisturiser
– SPF cream
– Reusable flannels or cloths

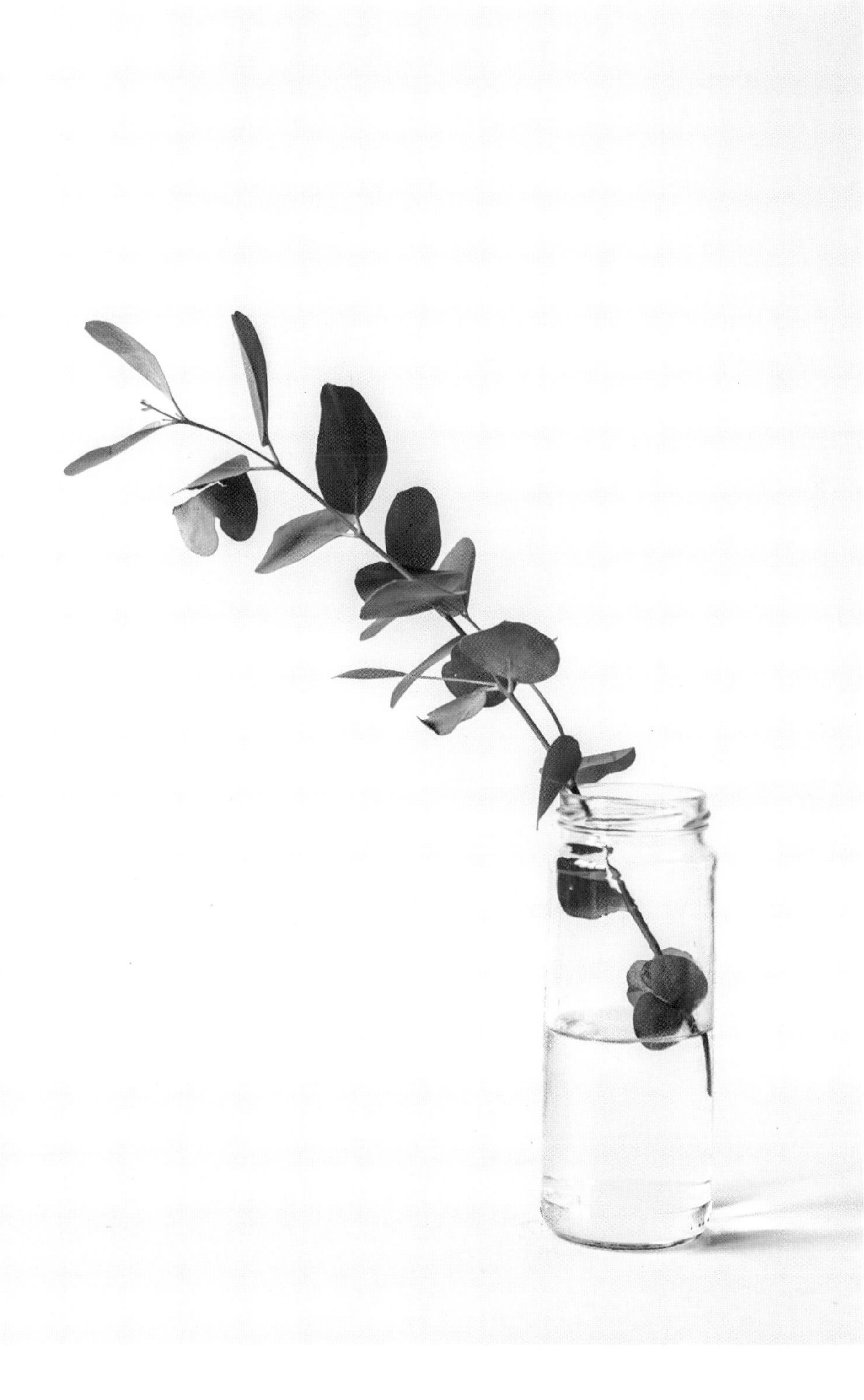

Magic all-purpose rescue balm

A good balm is a sustainable superhero in your bathroom cabinet. It can be used as a cleanser, moisturiser, make-up remover, overnight mask, dry skin treatment, cracked heel balm, hand treatment, lip balm, cuticle balm, brow tamer – and the list goes on. This recipe is my go-to rescue balm.

Makes 1 mask

Ingredients
– 2 tbsp rosehip oil
– 2 tbsp shea butter
– 1 tbsp candelilla wax
– 15 drops essential oil of your choice (optional)

Equipment
– Saucepan
– Heatproof glass or metal bowl (that sits snugly on top of the saucepan)
– Metal spoon
– Funnel
– Sterilised glass jar
– Heatproof gloves

Method
Fill the saucepan halfway with boiling water and set over a medium heat.

1. Place all the ingredients, apart from the essential oil, in the bowl.

2. Set the bowl over the saucepan and let the ingredients melt.

3. Once all the ingredients have completely melted, wearing heatproof gloves, remove the bowl carefully from the saucepan and place on a heatproof surface.

Wait 5 minutes for the balm to cool, then slowly add the essential oil, if using, stirring the whole time with the spoon. Mix well.

4. Once combined, use the funnel to pour the magic balm into the sterilised glass jar. Allow to cool for 1–2 hours.

5–6. While cooling, the balm will change colour and become thicker in texture. Store in a cool dark place for up to three months.

To apply, massage a coin-sized amount into the skin in a circular motion, concentrating on problem areas for congestion and dryness, like the nose. Massage into the skin for 2 minutes, then remove with a clean muslin or flannel.

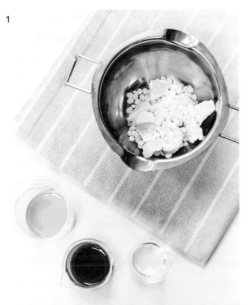

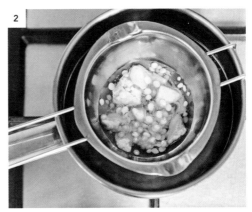

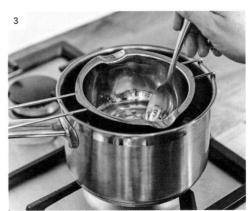

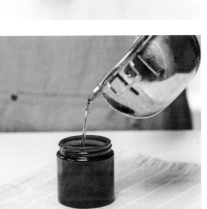

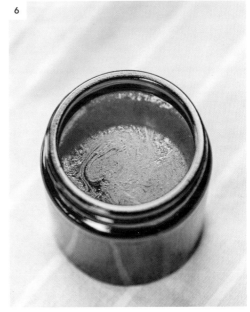

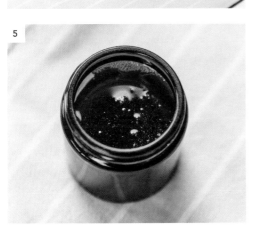

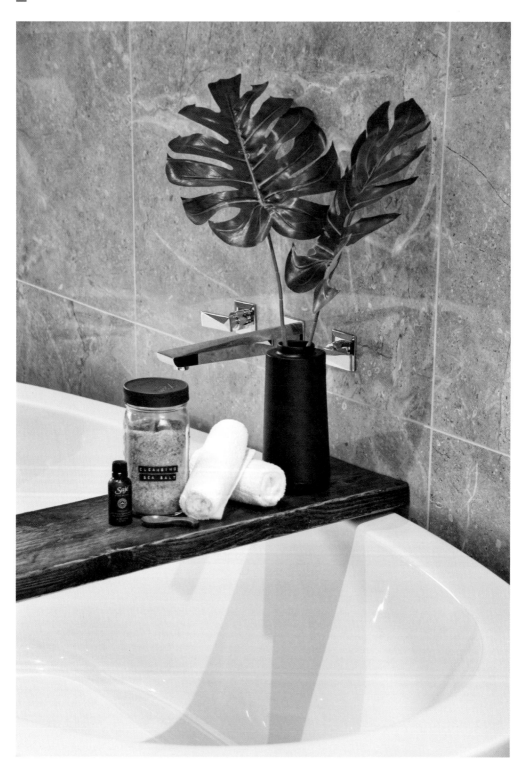

Bodycare
—

Antiperspirant vs deodorant

An antiperspirant works by blocking the sweating action of the glands, whereas a deodorant doesn't block the sweating process. Sweat is one of the ways your body detoxifies itself. There is a lot of debate about whether some of the ingredients in antiperspirants are carcinogenic. Studies have indicated that antiperspirants may be linked to breast or prostate cancer, however scientists have deemed them safe to use. I'm not a scientist, but perhaps whether they are safe needs further investigation; in either case I don't like the idea of blocking a detoxifying process. That just sounds like bad news to me.

Using a deodorant, you still sweat, but you won't smell. Sweat is odourless and odour occurs as a result of bacteria that lives on the skin, breaking down sweat into certain acids. Deodorants make the skin more acidic so that it's more difficult for the bacteria to grow. You will need to reapply deodorant throughout the day for it to be effective. Everybody's biochemistry is different, so you may need to try a few to find the one that works for you. Experiment by making your own (see page 75). Many deodorant recipes include bicarbonate of soda (baking soda), however it's an abrasive substance, so while it can work for other beauty products, it may irritate the delicate area under your arms.

Body washes and scrubs

Body washes are products that manufacturers love to stuff with foaming agents. In the INCI list you are likely to see sodium lauryl sulphate (SLS), amongst others. Swap to a plant-based body cleanser or consider using oils to cleanse your skin, much like you would your face. Oils are a fantastic body cleanser. Body bars are a good sustainable option as there is no requirement for excess packaging. Check they are not full of surfactants and fragrance like some traditional soaps, as these can dry out your skin.

Exfoliating products, such as body scrubs, have come under the microscope recently, due to the inclusion of microbeads in their formulation. Many countries have now banned microbeads from wash off products due to aquatic damage. These products instead use ingredients such as sugar, oats, jojoba seeds, walnut shells and salt for a similar effect. Consider a sustainable swap and invest in a dry brush to exfoliate your skin (see page 80).

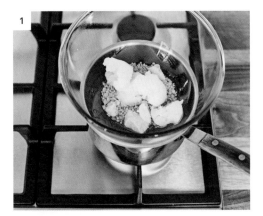

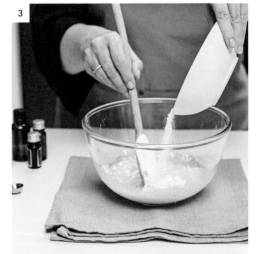

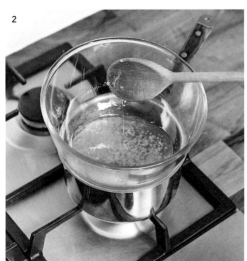

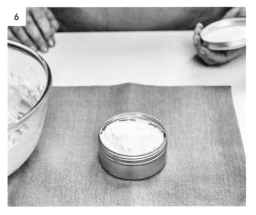

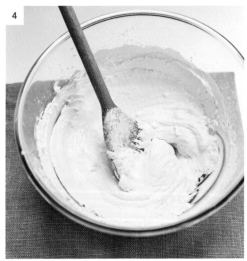

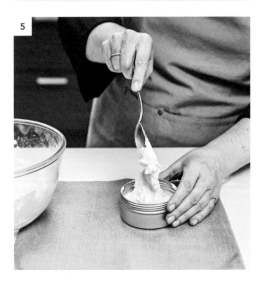

Arrowroot deodorant cream

Finding a natural deodorant that works for everybody is hard. After all, everyone's biochemistry is different, and has its own reaction to specific ingredients. That's why we tend to be disappointed when friends say they've found the Holy Grail of natural deodorants, but when we try it ourselves we smell like we've run a marathon. There is a transition period when swapping to a natural deodorant. You'll think it's not working, but stick with it until your body adjusts. After much research, I found this recipe. Let me know what you think!

Ingredients
- 4 tbsp virgin unrefined coconut oil
- 32g (1oz) candelilla wax
- 2 tbsp organic, unrefined shea butter
- ½ tsp vitamin E oil (optional)
- 85g (3oz) arrowroot powder
- 2 tbsp pharmaceutical grade, non-nano zinc oxide
- 15 drops lavender essential oil (optional)
- 10 drops cedarwood essential oil (optional)
- 5 drops vetiver essential oil (optional)

Equipment
- Heatproof glass bowl
- Wooden spoon
- Saucepan (make sure the glass bowl sits snugly on top)
- Reusable pot or jar with lid

Method

1. Place the coconut oil, shea butter and candelilla wax in the glass bowl.

2. Fill the saucepan halfway with water, place the pan on the hob over a medium heat and bring to a gentle simmer. Once simmering, place the glass bowl and mixture on top of the saucepan and gently heat for a few minutes until melted, stirring occasionally with the wooden spoon.

3. Turn off the heat and remove the bowl. Add the vitamin E oil (if using), arrowroot and zinc oxide, stirring continuously.

4. Leave to cool for a minute or two, then add the essential oils (if using).

5–6. Immediately scoop the mixture into a wide-necked pot or jar and seal it with a lid. Store in a cool dark place.

To use, take a small amount and rub it between your fingers. Massage this onto your armpit and leave to dry for a few seconds. Repeat with other armpit.

A healing oat soak for sensitive skin

Oats are pretty wonderful. Not only are they great for the nervous system (yes, your porridge can help with anxiety), they are also an excellent skin soother, softener and cleanser. They contain calcium, iron and vitamin B1 and are natural antioxidants. If you have very sensitive skin, oats are an effective alternative to soaps and detergents. This super quick recipe for creating a healing oat bath bag is one you can do with your family, and it also makes a gorgeous gift.

Ingredients
–   A large handful of
    organic oats
–   A small handful of dried
    lavender flowers (omit
    these if you have very
    sensitive skin)

Equipment
–   Food processor
–   A square of muslin
    (cheesecloth)
–   A repurposed rubber
    band or hair band
–   Twine or repurposed
    white or cream ribbon

Method
1–2. Place the oats into a food processor. If you wish, you can add in a small handful of dried lavender flowers. (These will make your oat bag smell incredible and have a calming and relaxing effect.) Blend to a fine powder.

3. Lay a square of muslin on a flat surface and tip the mixture into the centre.

4–5. Gather the edges of the fabric into a central point and hold tightly just above the mound of oat powder. Take a rubber band or hair band and secure the cloth.

6. Cover it with twine or repurposed ribbon.

To use, run a bath, placing the oat bag under the tap and letting the properties of the oats soak into the water. Gently squeeze the bag and the water will turn cloudy. Sink back into the warm bath, take a few deep breaths and relax. Use the oat bag as a body cleanser; the muslin cloth will act as a gentle exfoliator. When you have finished, the oat mixture can be composted and the muslin washed and reused.

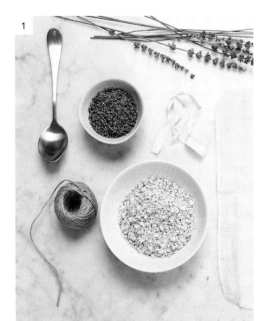

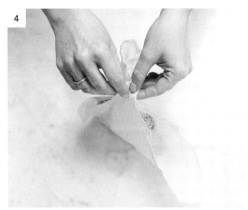

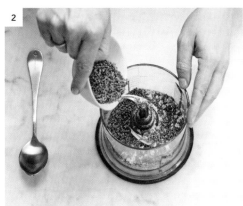

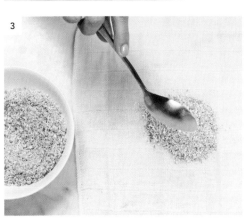

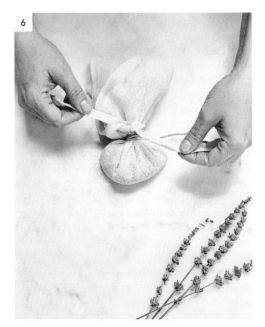

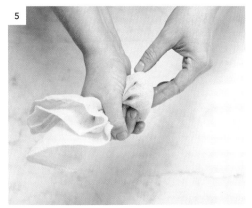

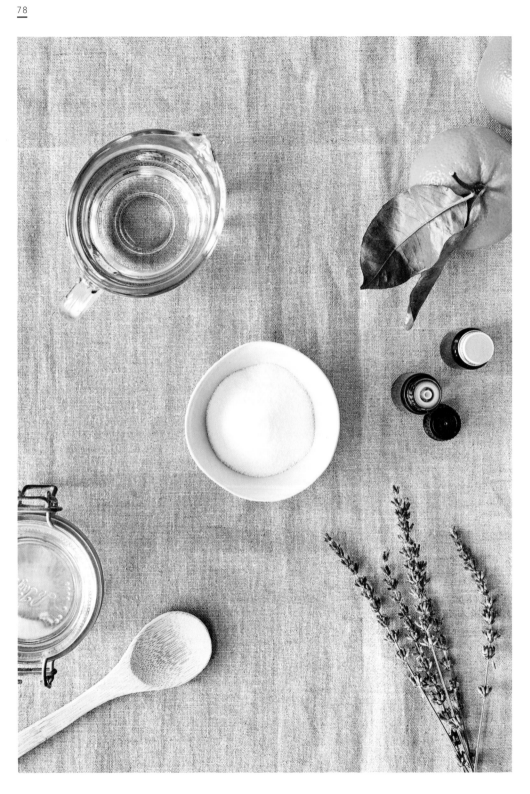

Night-time body scrubs

Not only do body scrubs slough off old skin, but they also buff, polish and moisturise. There's something evocative about the scent conjured by marrying the deliciously dry and earthy sandalwood with the dreamy, soothing notes of rose – they just work! I know rose oil isn't cheap – but it's amazing! It's a natural antidepressant, calming and uplifting for the spirit. It also strengthens tissue and is antibacterial, moisturising, antiviral and anti-ageing! A dreamy mandarin and lavender oil mix is perfect to use just before you go to bed, helping you relax and be calm. Keep a jar beside the bath and use liberally whenever you want to pamper yourself.

Ingredients

Rose, salt and sandalwood
- 64g (2¼oz/¼ cup) sea salt
- 240ml (8fl oz/1 cup) fractionated (liquid) or melted coconut oil
- 4–5 drops pure rose essential oil
- 4–5 drops sandalwood essential oil

Mandarin and lavendar
- 64g (2¼oz/¼ cup) sea salt
- 240ml (8fl oz/1 cup) fractionated (liquid) or melted coconut oil
- 6 drops mandarin essential oil
- 4 drops lavender essential oil

Equipment
- Mixing bowl
- Wooden spoon
- Repurposed glass jar with lid, sterilised

Method

1. In the mixing bowl, stir together the salt and the coconut oil.

2. Add the essential oils to the mix, blending well. Transfer to a glass jar to store.

To use, take a scoop and rub gently onto wet skin using slow, circular movements, then rinse off.

Dry brushing

Invest in a good dry brush and you'll never need a body exfoliant again. Dry brushing is so good for the skin, increases blood flow and detoxifies by promoting lymph flow drainage. Look out for vegan bristles and a sustainable wood or bamboo handle. Dry brushing is a better alternative to using cellulite creams.

TECHNIQUE: Use once or twice a week before bathing or, if you have super sensitive skin, just a couple of times per month. Start at the soles of your feet and, using long strokes, brush up your legs on to your buttocks. Then start at your hands and brush up your arms toward your shoulders. Brush your chest and back in shorter strokes always toward the heart and in a circular motion over your abdomen. It can feel strange at first, but then you start to love the invigorating feeling. Afterward, jump in the shower or bath and wash off the dead skin cells. Dry brushing helps with eliminating toxins so is a useful technique for cellulite. Wash your brush regularly to remove dead skin cells.

Body lotions, creams, butters and oils

Here you can really relish in the benefits of wonderful natural ingredients such as shea butter, cocoa butter, mango butter, jojoba oil and coconut oil. In terms of richness, a lotion is the lightest in texture and a body butter is the richest. Use your body product over your bust; you do not need a separate product.

Body lotions and creams are made from mixing oil and water. The thickness of the product depends on the ratio used. Both are effective at keeping skin hydrated and moisturized. Body lotions are a good all-round option; their higher water content means they are simple to apply, absorb more easily into the skin, and are readily available. Because they are quickly absorbed, they are useful if you need to dress immediately after. Lotions are also a good option for people with body acne, excessive sweating and psoriasis. Sensitive skins should avoid fragranced lotions. Creams are thicker and more soothing for dry skin, but can have a greasier residue, so are best used when you have more time for the product to fully absorb into the skin.

Body oils are great to seal in moisture and reinforce the skin's barrier layer. Oily skin also responds well to oils, as they balance the skin and reduce its tendency to over-produce its own oil. Instantly soothing and easy to apply, you will have an slippery feel to the skin straight after, so choose a different product if you need to dress immediately; if you have time allow it to absorb, you'll be left with a gorgeous sheen. Oils will only affect the surface of the skin as opposed to other products like lotions, which will penetrate deeper.

Body butters have a high vitamin content and are amazing to soothe and soften rough, itchy and dry skin patches, like elbows, feet, heels and hands. Massage in until the product is absorbed completely. Consistent use will give you the most hydrated and soft skin. It's super easy to make your own butter – follow my nourishing rose souffle body butter for dry skin recipe on page 82. A multi-use product, you can also use this butter on your face and as a lip balm.

Remember that it's not only food oils and fats that cause fatberg blockages in our sewers and drains, which is why it's so important to dispose of any beauty `products containing these ingredients in your rubbish and not down your sinks.

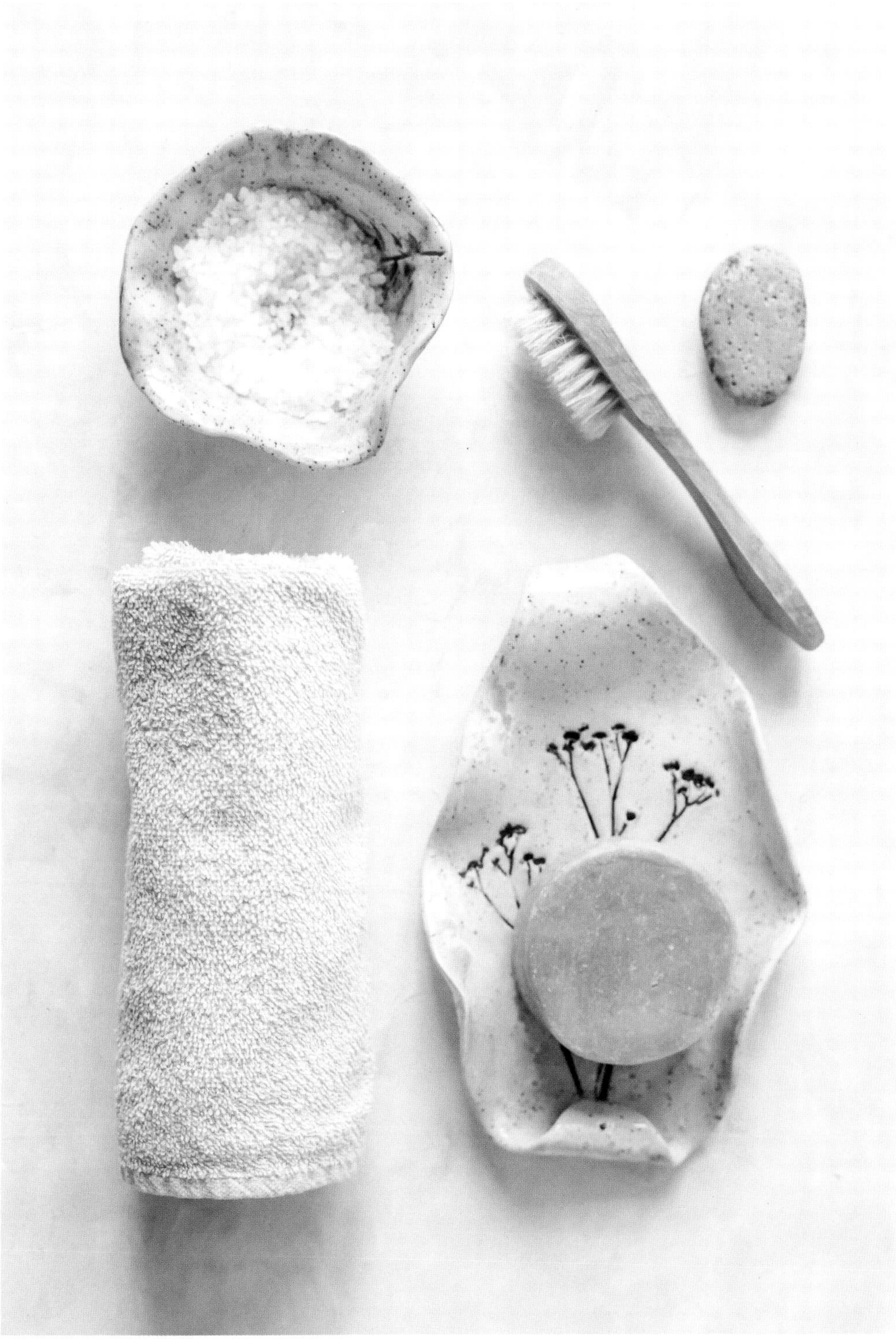

Nourishing rose soufflé body butter for dry skin

Suitable for anyone, of any age, with dry skin, this cloud-soft skin soufflé is a total treat. This takes a little more time than some of the other recipes, but boy is it worth it! It offers lasting hydration and deep moisturising, along with conditioning and skin-smoothing properties. You can apply it direct from the jar to face or body. Any leftovers can be immersed in a bath (ensuring the water is not too hot – test before hopping in). Once the butter has melted, it will form a film on the surface of the bath water. Relax in your bath, and when you emerge, the butter and oils will have adhered to your skin and hair. Take time to massage in for a full-strength softening treatment. For dry feet, apply a generous amount before bed and wear cotton socks to sleep in. This butter is so good you'll want to eat it! Your skin will never have felt so soft!

Note: As with any oil treatment, please use towels on the floor to prevent slipping.

Ingredients
- 70g (2½oz) shea butter
- 70g (2½oz) cocoa butter
- 5 tbsp coconut oil
- 1 tbsp vitamin E oil
- 5 drops rose essential oil
- 3 drops frankincense essential oil

Equipment
- Saucepan
- Heatproof glass bowl
- (that sits snugly on top
- of the saucepan)
- Electric whisk/balloon whisk
- Wooden spoon
- Spatula
- Clean repurposed jar, or similar container, sterilised

Method
Heat about one quarter of a saucepan of water over a high heat. Once boiling, reduce the heat to a gentle simmer.

1. Place the shea butter, cocoa butter, coconut oil and vitamin E oil into the glass bowl and place on top of the simmering saucepan, or use a bain marie. After 5 minutes the mixture should be liquified and have combined.

2. Using heat-proof gloves, carefully remove the bowl from the saucepan. Leave to cool for a minute, then add the essential oils and mix with the spoon.

3. Place the glass bowl in the freezer for 15 minutes (or until 70 per cent of the mixture is solid but still soft).

4. Whisk for about 5 minutes, or until the mixture is light and fluffy. If whisking by hand with a balloon whisk, this may take longer.

5–6. Using a spatula, scrape the mixture out of the bowl and transfer it to a repurposed jar with a lid and seal.

To apply, take a small amount and massage it into the skin using circular movements.

1

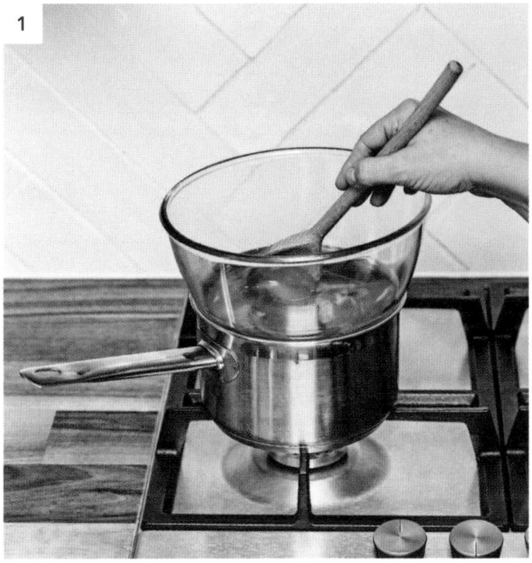

2

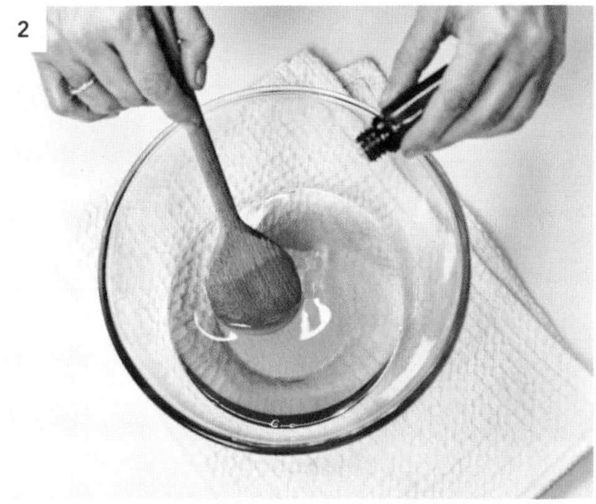

3

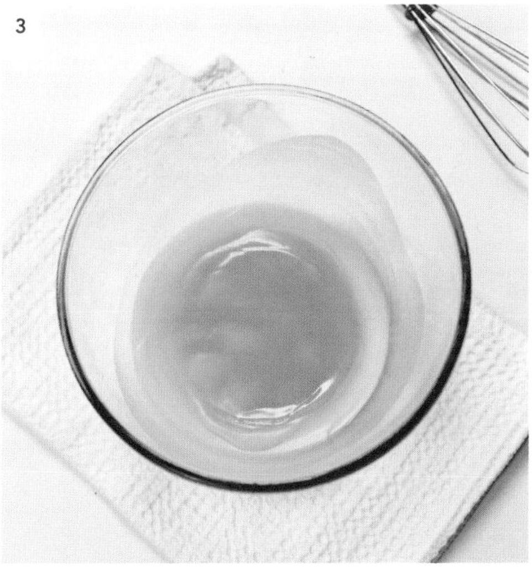

4

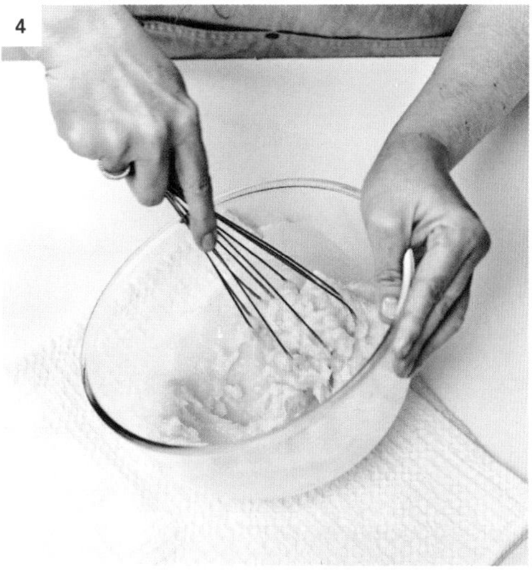

5

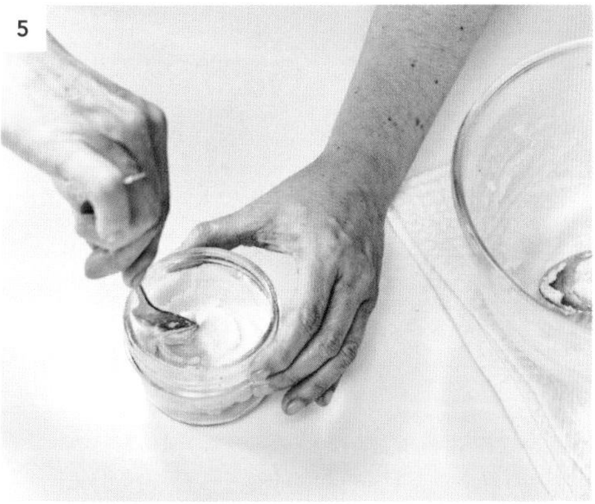

6

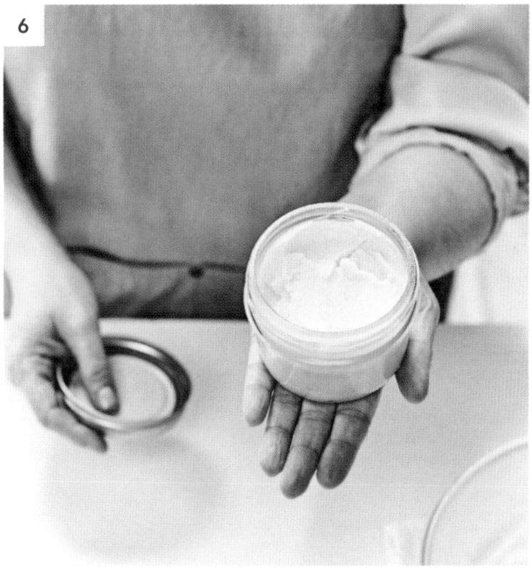

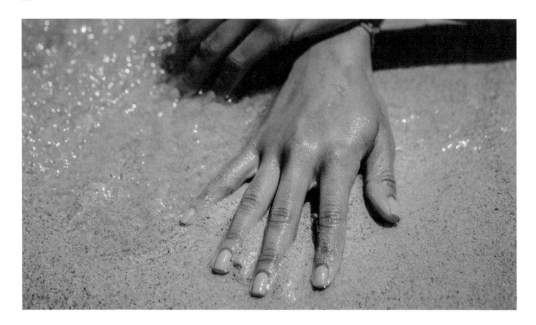

Hands, feet and nails

Your hands and feet are constantly working, yet they are often neglected when it comes to self-care. Something as simple as moisturising your hands a couple of times a day can make all the difference and prevent your hands from feeling sore and dry. Body lotion is perfect to use on hands and feet, and if you need something richer, try the rose souffle body butter on page 82 . A great balm will keep cuticles soft, prevent any splits and will keep heels from cracking. Don't forget the cuticles on your toes too. The magic all-purpose rescue balm on page 70 is ideal. Alternatively, an oil works perfectly to keep cuticles supple. A foot scrub once a week will keep the skin smooth and get rid of any dead skin cells that can cause dryness. For an easy quick scrub recipe, try the rose, salt and sandalwood body scrub on page 78.

You'll need some other tools to keep hands and feet healthy. A good-quality pair of toenail clippers will make light of a tricky job. If you can invest in the best your budget allows, they'll last forever and you'll find they will perform a better, cleaner cut, thus preventing ingrown nails. The same goes for nail scissors. If your toenails are particularly brittle, cut them after a bath, or immerse your feet for 10 minutes in the rosemary and tea tree foot soak recipe on page 88. An old-school pumice stone is handy to keep in your bathroom cupboard. Rub the stone over areas of hard skin, then rinse in water to clean. An orange stick is useful to push back cuticles and a glass nail file will keep your nails groomed. A glass file is long lasting and if it's plain with no embellishments, it can simply be recycled in your recycling bin at the end of its life.

Prevention is better than cure, but if you already have hard skin and cracked heels, develop a daily routine and you'll see improvements. Regular use of a pumice stone and foot scrub, along with daily use of a lotion and balm, will work wonders. For sore and dry hands, at night apply moisturiser followed by a thick layer of balm. In the morning, your hands will feel smooth and hydrated.

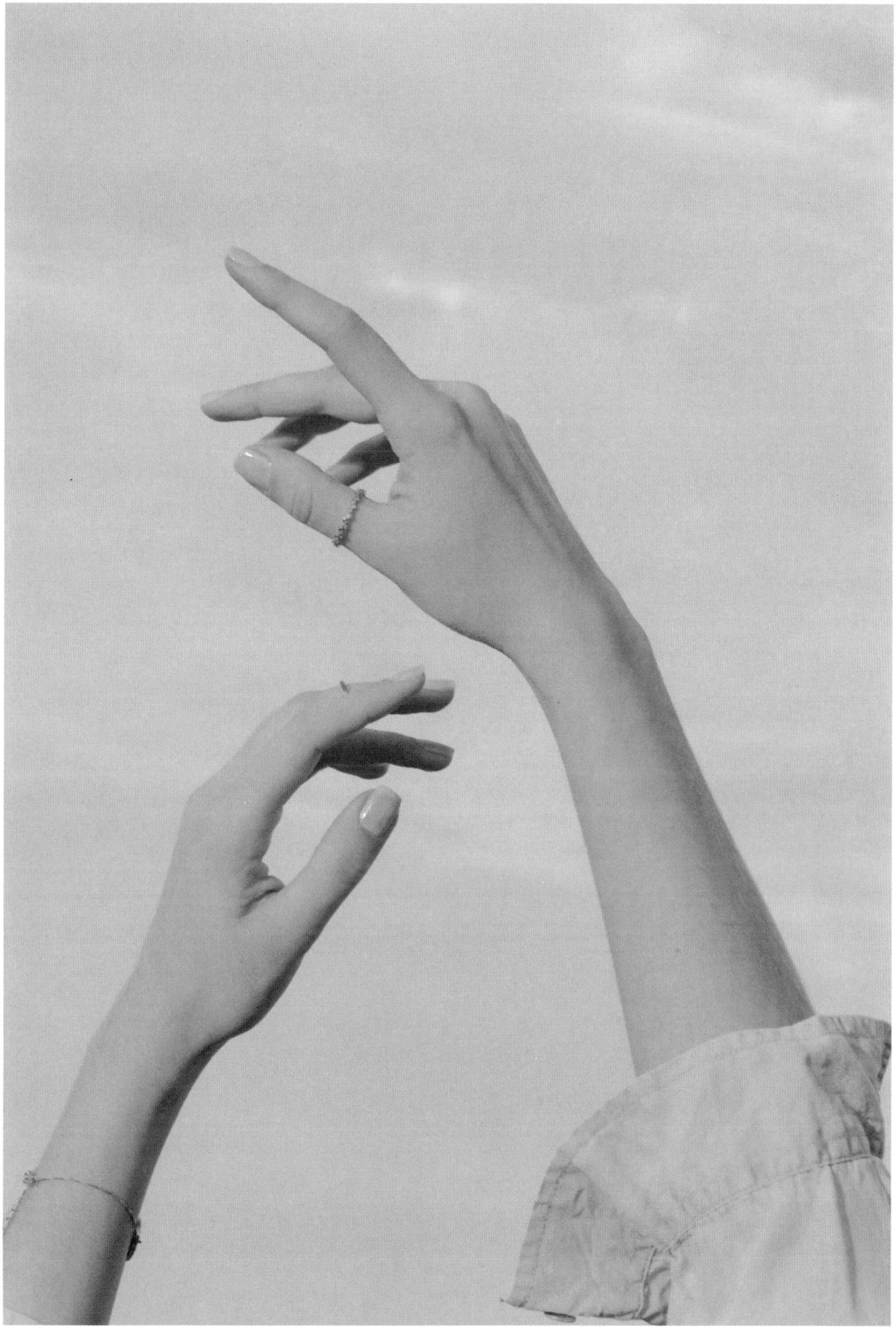

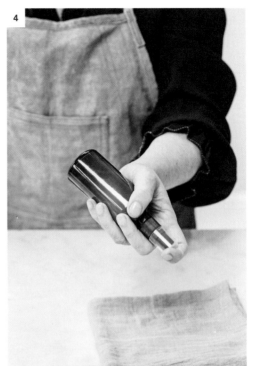

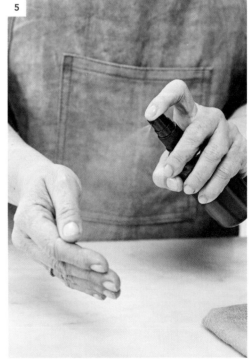

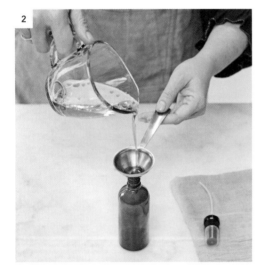

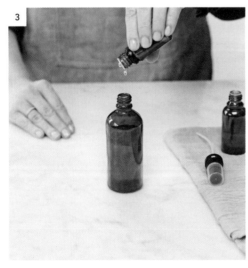

Vodka and grapefruit, holiday cocktail, hand sanitiser

Our world is now awash with hand sanitiser at every turn. Many of them are full of the wrong types of chemicals, toxic oddities and alcohol – cruel, but necessary when it comes to bacteria-bashing! My recipe blends grain alcohol (ethanol) with a high-proof vodka (don't judge me) and a peppering of grapefruit essential oil. It smells like a holiday cocktail – hence the name – and the best thing is, it works!

The alcohol and the tea tree oil, which I also include, kill bacteria, while the vitamin E serves to moisturise the skin. Meanwhile, the grapefruit adds a zesty scent, as well as being antibacterial and antimicrobial. It's good to remember that nothing is quite like good old-fashioned soap and hot water to sanitise your hands, but when you're on the move, this is my go-to product. An added bonus is that it costs a fraction of the price of a shop-bought version, which may have additives.

Ingredients

– 60ml (2fl oz/¼ cup) ethanol alcohol
– 2 tsp vodka (whichever brand you might have lingering in the cupboards)
– 7 drops tea tree essential oil
– 5 drops grapefruit essential oil
– 20ml (²/₃fl oz/4 tsp) vitamin E oil

Equipment

– Measuring jug
– Small funnel
– 100ml (3½fl oz) repurposed glass bottle with pump dispenser, sterilised

Method

1. Measure out the necessary amounts of ethanal and vodka into the jug.

2. Place the funnel into the bottle and pour the ethanol–vodka mix in.

3–4. Add in the essential oils and vitamin E oil. Seal with the pump dispenser top and shake well.

5. To use, spritz.

Rosemary and tea tree foot soak

Submerging tired feet into this cleansing and moisturising foot soak feels almost ritualistic! Puffiness and soreness slip away as the rosemary oil offers a leafy, zesty scent and the tea tree provides antibacterial properties. The oils soften and soothe, while the salts slough off dead skin. The rosemary oil is also an effective mood enhancer. If you have a rosemary plant in your house or garden, snip off a few stems. Place into a mug with hot water and, while you soak your feet, take some deep breaths and sip slowly for an anti-inflammatory, antimicrobial and antioxidant warming tea.

Ingredients

- 240ml (8fl oz/1 cup) fractionated (liquid) or melted coconut oil
- 120ml (4fl oz/½ cup) olive oil (not extra virgin)
- 10 drops rosemary essential oil
- 5 drops tea tree essential oil
- 1 tbsp Epsom salts (optional)
- Handful of sea salt
- Large bowl warm water, for the foot bath

Equipment

- Mixing bowl
- Metal spoon/metal whisk
- 225ml (8fl oz) repurposed glass container/jam jar with lid, sterilised

Method

1. Pour the melted coconut oil into the mixing bowl. Add the olive oil and whisk together.

2–3. Add the essential oils and the salt. Mix well with the spoon, or ideally whisk until combined.

4. Pour the mixture into the jar and wait for contents to settle.

5. To use, scoop a few tablespoons of the foot soak into the large bowl of warm water, stirring well. Sit back and soak your feet in the warm healing waters. Bliss!

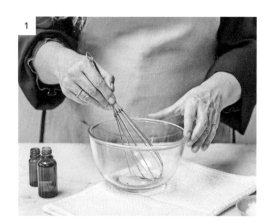

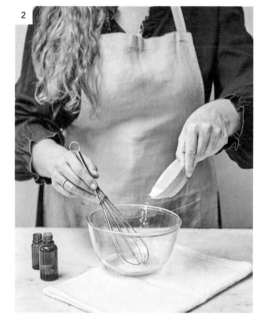

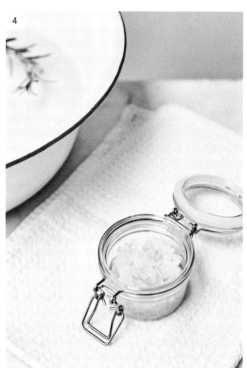

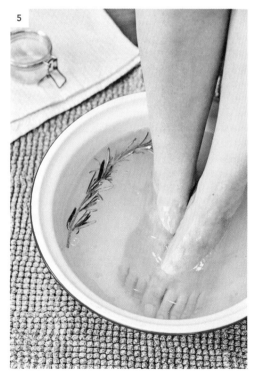

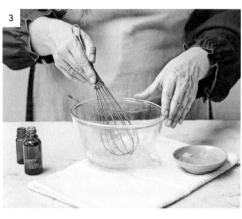

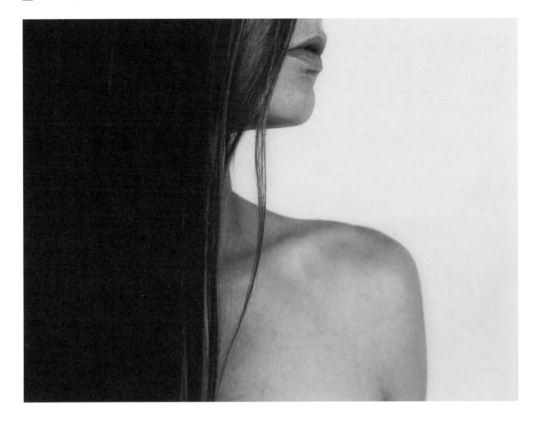

Haircare

—

Conserving water

Believe it or not, continuously washing your hair isn't the best option for hair health. It's also not the healthiest option for the environment due to the amount of water used and the chemicals in our hair products draining away down the plug hole. Try washing your hair less. Your hair will adjust. For those days just before your next wash, hair scarves, bands and wraps are useful accessories, and a natural dry shampoo is also great for absorbing oil in between washes.

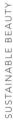

Hair cleansing

Co-washing

Co-washing is a technique whereby you use a cleansing conditioner to wash your hair. Many people with dry, wavy, Afro, curly, coarse or colour-treated hair swear by it. You are basically cleaning your hair with a conditioner that has extra cleansing ingredients added.

Why do it? Most shampoos are formulated with sulphates, which are foaming agents that make us feel psychologically that we are cleaning our hair properly. In fact, these ingredients dry out the hair and scalp, so too much washing can impair your hair health. Cleansing conditioners allow natural oils to clean, nourish and hydrate the hair and scalp. For best results, choose co-washing products that are silicone-free. One word of caution: always use a product labelled as a 'co-wash'. This will ensure it contains the right balance of cleansing ingredients, so that you can ensure dirt is still lifted from your hair and scalp. Do not just use your conditioner as a shampoo, otherwise your hair may not feel clean but heavy and laden with product.

Shampoo

To maintain healthy hair, it's important to use shampoos that are sulphate-free. They won't foam up as much as your traditional shampoos, but you don't need foam to clean, and they will be much kinder to your hair. Shampoo bars are a great option to reduce packaging. Again, look for plant-based bars and ones in FSC-certified paper and cardboard packaging.

Focus on naturally cleansing and antiseptic ingredients such as tea tree oil and eucalyptus. Coconut oil and witch hazel are great for shine and condition. However, if you have low porosity hair, coconut oil can dry out your hair, so look for lighter oil ingredients such as fractionated coconut oil, jojoba, argan and sweet almond oil. If you have oily hair, over-washing isn't the answer; you need to wash your hair and scalp to remove

the oil, but not so much that the scalp feels stripped and produces more oil. Experiment with how often you wash your hair to work out what is best for you. If you find it too difficult to cut down on washing your hair, it's even more important that you use botanicals (plant-based ingredients), not just to help cleanse and nourish the hair in a gentler way, but to be more sustainable, as whatever ingredients we use to wash our hair goes down the plug hole and drains into our sewers and waterways.

Dry shampoo

This product has been around since the 1940s – Twiggy even appeared in an ad for one in the 1960s. It's basically a powder formulation that disguises excess oil in the hair. Usually in a powder shaker container or an aerosol spray, it's excellent for extending the time between hair washes. Avoid commercial products, as overuse can lead to dry hair and scalp. A much better option is to choose one with naturally derived ingredients like arrowroot powder.

Hair nourishing

If you have chemically treated, Afro, curly, coloured or damaged hair, it's even more important to nourish your hair. Try to avoid those quick-fix ingredients. Surfactants and silicones, which will bring instant relief and shine but will not support long-term hair health.

Conditioner

If you colour your hair like me, you know the feeling when the conditioner eventually goes on – you breathe a sigh of relief that your hair hasn't actually turned into a matted rug, and all is well again in hair world. Commercial conditioners immediately make your hair feel smooth and silky, but unfortunately they contain silicones and surfactants, which are not good for your long-term hair health or the environment. The good news is that there is an abundance of plant-based conditioners, packed full of nourishing, eco-friendly botanicals.

Deep conditioning is a more intense form of conditioning, which benefits all hair types once a week or every fortnight. After applying, wear your shower cap and leave for 30–45 minutes before washing off.

Leave-in treatments

Particularly effective on dry, damaged, colour-treated, curly or Afro hair, the right leave-in products can provide extra moisture and protection, and add shine and strength. Make sure your leave-in products are full of naturally derived plant-based ingredients and are silicone-free.

The ingredients and methods of application you choose become paramount if you have high or low porosity hair. High porosity hair absorbs water, oils and other ingredients easily, however it doesn't retain moisture well. Low porosity hair, on the other hand, does not easily absorb moisture

and tends to repel it. If it takes ages for your hair to get saturated with water when washing it, you are likely to have low porosity hair. High porosity hair often feels dry no matter how much product you add. Both hair types will love the hair healing rinse recipe on page 101. It will gently clarify low porosity hair and, if used as a finishing treatment, will close the cuticles of high porosity hair.

Hair mask

Hair masks work on exactly the same principle as a face mask – giving an extra boost of whatever your hair needs. A once-a-week treatment can be beneficial, as long as the ingredients serve your long-term hair health. Overuse of commercial hair masks can result in limp and dull hair due to the inclusion of silicones and surfactants. If you make a sustainable swap from commercial shampoos and conditioners, you might find the condition of your hair improves so you don't need a separate hair mask. If you do need a treatment, use natural oils and wrap your hair in a hot towel, or make the Mexican hair mask (see page 94).

TECHNIQUES AND INGREDIENTS:

High porosity hair: try the LOC method, which is applying liquid, oil, cream in that order. The liquid is water and will give the hair moisture. Hair doesn't need to be soaking wet, but make sure it is the wetter side of damp so the following products work more effectively. Section the hair to apply water and treatments so that each strand is coated. Next add oils such as jojoba or sweet almond. Depending on personal preference, you can add the oil all over or just to the end lengths. Finally add a cream or butter; shea, mango or cocoa butter work well for some hair types but if they are too rich for you, stick to a cream. If you like butters, whip them up so they are lighter to use. You can also try swapping the order, so after liquid, apply cream first, then oil. Experiment to see what is best for your hair.

Low porosity hair can also benefit from the LOC or LCO system, but the water used should be warm to open up the cuticle. Apply your conditioning treatments and leave-in products alongside heat, so that the cuticles lift and moisture can be absorbed. Hot towels, steam and a shower cap (called the 'greenhouse effect') are useful methods to use. Oils such as sweet almond, argan, jojoba, fractionated coconut oil and grapeseed work well. For a midweek boost, add some aloe vera concentrate to water and spritz over the hair.

For all hair types, always use a wide-tooth comb!

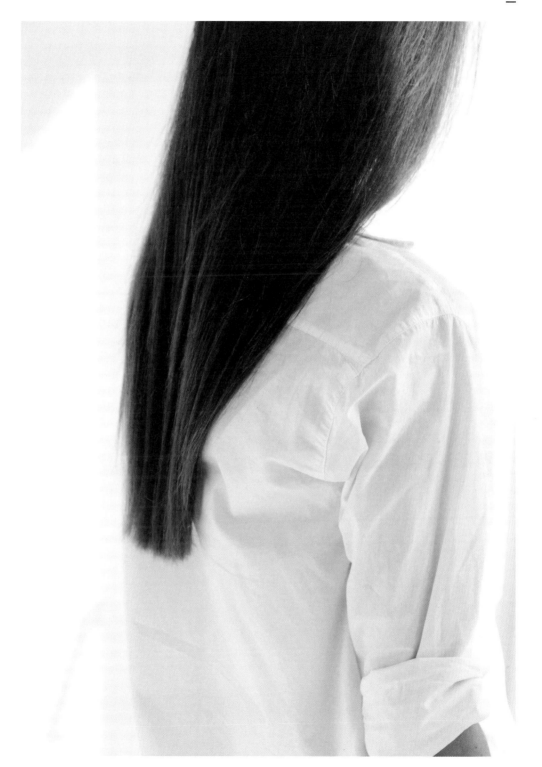

Mexican hair mask

About 10 years ago, my partner and I were on holiday in Mexico. We were staying in a gorgeous eco-boutique beach hotel on the Yucatán Peninsula. The owner provided handmade bathroom goodies. Among them was a fabulous hair mask. It was like a gloriously gloopy cocktail for your hair – surely everything is right about that? I'm not below begging and that's pretty much what I had to do to get this recipe. In this unequal exchange, the quantities were not revealed, so I've had to practice, adapt and add to it to get it right. But the results were worth it. While you are waiting for the mask to conjure up its magic, add a spoonful of apple cider vinegar to hot water as a tea and drink to enjoy its amazing all-round health benefits.

Makes: 1–3 applications (depending on hair length)

Ingredients
- 4 tbsp agave nectar
- 2 tbsp apple cider vinegar
- 1 tbsp fractionated (liquid) or melted coconut oil
- ½ tbsp olive oil
- Squeeze of lime juice (half a lime)
- 3 drops ylang ylang essential oil

Equipment
- Clean glass jar with a lid, sterilised

Method

1–3. Decant all the ingredients into the jar, seal with a lid and shake vigorously.

To use, apply a handful of the gloopy tonic generously to damp or wet hair, massaging into the scalp. Then comb through.

Leave for a minimum of 15 minutes.

Rinse with lukewarm water. Dry and style hair.

Shampoo as normal.

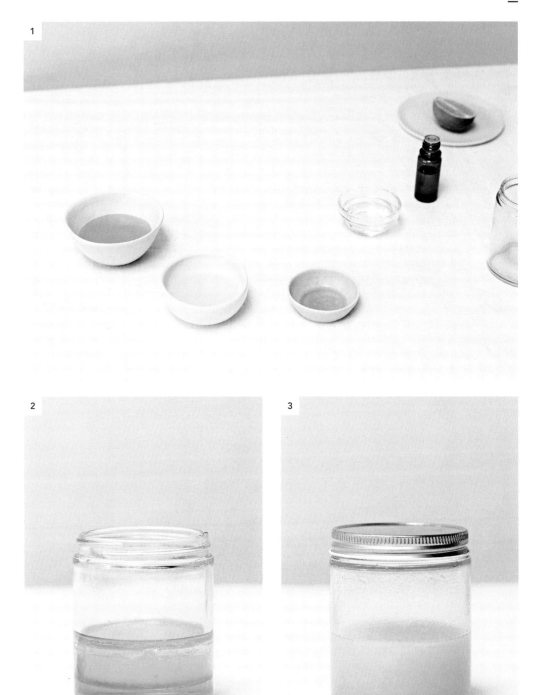

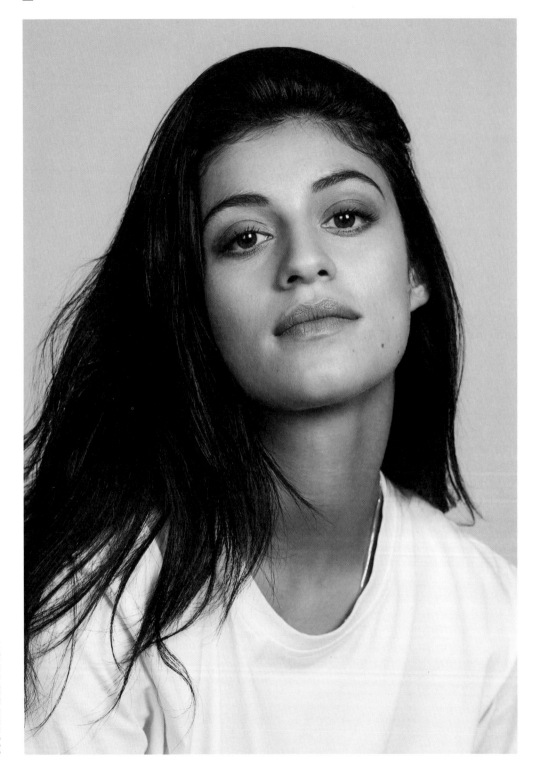

Hair styling

The healthiest way to style your hair for long-term health is without heat, however not many of us can do that. There are ways you can be more mindful, reduce damage to your hair and use less energy. If you wash and blow-dry your hair every day, consider spritzing it with water on subsequent days, combing through and re-styling, rather than completely washing your hair all over again. If you use styling products with more plant-based ingredients, you will have less build-up on the hair, and less of a need to constantly wash it. Consider air-drying your hair, or if you must blow-dry, then wait until it's 75 per cent air-dried before blasting it with the hairdryer. Once you have used your hairdryer on a section of hair, use the cooling button, if it has one. This will lock in the style, so should save you having to redo your styling to the same extent the next day.

Air-drying, root lift and hemp towels

Air-drying your hair uses less energy and is also healthier for your hair. Root lift is important to many styles, but it can be a challenge when air-drying due to the weight of wet hair. Use a hemp towel to gently squeeze the hair to absorb excess moisture. Don't wring your hair or rub it, as this can create frizz and breakage, especially for curly, textured or colour-treated hair. Hemp towels are more sustainable than cotton or microfibre towels. Tip your head upside down every now and then and massage the roots gently. This will encourage the hair to lift up rather than be dragged down. If you have long hair, pin up the ends to reduce the weight until the crown is nearly dry, then release the ends to dry too. Pin your hair up in twists, braids or pin curls, as this is a good way to get a bit of movement and wave in straighter hair, and to capture the curl in curly or textured hair. For tousled hair, apply an oil or cream product, or both, when it is damp. Then every now and then, until the hair is 75 per cent dry, cup the ends of the hair in your hand then scrunch and lift in an upwards motion. To air dry Afro hair use the L.O.C method on damp, not wet

Microfibre towels have become very popular in recent years due to the amount of water they absorb, and they do not damage weak hair. A word of caution however. Every time a synthetic material like microfibre is washed, it releases microplastics into our waterways, which can end up in our rivers and seas, damaging marine life. If you do purchase one, make sure it's from a reputable company that uses better-quality microfibre that doesn't break up easily. Cheaper brands won't be made to last.

Styling products

Styling mousse and gel

Mousse has been around for decades. It comes in and out of fashion, but anyone with curly hair will be familiar with mousse. I remember having quite crispy curls at some points in the '80s and thought that I was the bee's knees. Mousse is designed to be a quick-drying product, and any quick-drying product will contain high volumes of alcohol, even plant-based products. The issue with alcohols that enable a product to be quick-drying is that they remove moisture from the hair. Overuse of this styling product can dry out and damage the hair, so limit its use or make a sustainable swap out and use a plant-based, alcohol-free styling lotion instead. You can recycle mousse cans, but make sure they are empty and that any plastic tops have been removed.

Gel is another option. There are so many on the market, from watery consistency light-hold gels to thick, heavy gels designed to make the hair rock hard. Look for a lightweight plant-based gel that is alcohol- and silicone-free so it won't dry out your hair.

Setting lotion

These are the lotions that our grandmothers and great-grandmothers used in the '40s to set their hair into waves and victory rolls. They are amazing for giving the hair a wave that will not budge, but boy do they dry out the hair. The alcohol content is off the scale; sniff the bottle and you'll know what I mean. Unless you are going to a '40s revival night, don't go near these if you want to retain lustrous locks.

Curl cream

A lightweight cream is a must for curly or Afro hair. Look for products containing oils such as flaxseed, which improves hair elasticity. Creams work well at conditioning hair, but are not a replacement for conditioners themselves, as they only work on the outside of the strands. Creams layer well with oil and gel products. When using with oil products they can be applied before or after, but with gel products they need to be applied beforehand.

> **TECHNIQUE:** Apply to wet rather than damp hair in order to capture the curl. Work in small sections. Rub a small amount between your palms and begin with the mid-sections, working the product down to the ends of the hair. What is left on your hands can be applied to your roots and your crown section. Working in small amounts allows you to see how much of a particular product you require. It's easier to add rather than try to remove product, and prevents any wastage.

Hairspray

A typical commercial hairspray contains polymers (chain-like molecules) in a solvent, a propellant, alcohol and fragrance; some contain essential oils. The plastic polymers wrap around the hair shaft, creating a stiff coating that prevents styles from dropping out. There are natural hairsprays out there that include more moisturising ingredients to offset the drying effects of a high alcohol content. Some brands use pump sprays, instead of aerosols, which negates the need for a chemical propellant.

If you have a natural hairstyle and don't need huge amounts of staying power, then consider doing a sustainable swap out and use a balm to tame any flyways instead of hairspray. The balm you use will need to be hard, not soft. Lip balm is a good texture to go on – the harder ones rather than the greasy ones. Either apply to the hair directly, or take an old blusher or powder make-up brush that you no longer use, wipe over the balm then apply in gentle sweeps over the hair. My vegan lip balm on page 139 works well to tame stray hairs.

Heat protection products

Heat is damaging to the hair, so every time you use your hairdryer, flat irons, heated rollers or tongs, it's important to redress and offset that damage. Heat protection products are designed to do just that. However, there's a dilemma. The majority of heat protection products on the market contain silicones which coat the hair in a plastic-like film. This film protects it from heat damage, but does not allow the hair to absorb moisture and nutrients. If it's not removed with a clarifying shampoo, which in itself strips the hair, the long-term effect is limp, dull, lifeless hair. So if you can, avoid heat. Use air-drying techniques and limit the heat you use. Choose gentler, naturally derived heat protection ingredients such as coconut, argan or grapeseed oil, shea butter and almond oil.

> **TECHNIQUE:** When using a natural oil, only a few drops are required. Section your hair, and rub the oil or product between your hands. Start at the mid-section and work down to the ends of your hair. Press the small amount of product left on your hands around the top of your head, avoiding your roots. This will stop your hair looking too greasy.

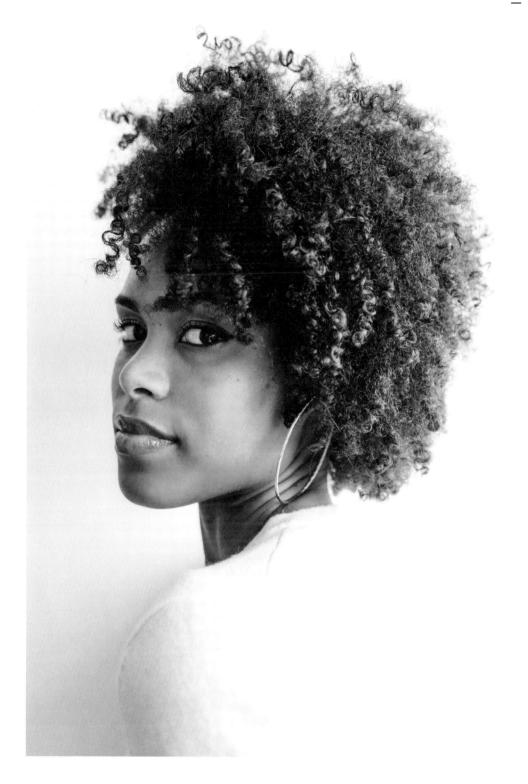

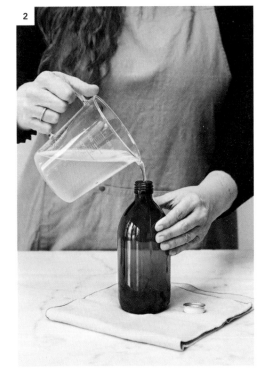

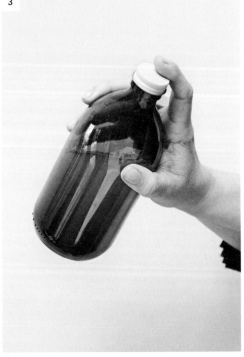

Hair healing rinse

The key ingredient in my herb-oil-infused hair rinse is raw apple cider vinegar –
aka ACV. Apple cider vinegar has been used for yonks in both cooking and, for its
medicinal properties, home remedies. Not everybody knows that this incredible
ingredient is bursting with brilliant hair-care properties too. Among them are that it
cleanses (ACV is antibacterial) and exfoliates the scalp, hydrates and softens, as well
as giving a healthy sheen to the hair.

In this recipe, I also added rosemary and clary sage essential oils which, between
them, thicken and strengthen the hair. I make enough for a week or two and decant
it into a repurposed spray/vaporizer bottle or a jar. After shampooing, simply apply
the mixture to the hair and leave for three minutes, but if you are pushed for time,
this even works after a minute. Remember that ACV is a vinegar, so be cautious if you
have any cuts or grazes on your hands or scalp when using this, as it could sting and
cause redness. I love this recipe; it's so easy, cost effective and it works.

**Makes: 1–2 applications
(depending on hair length)**

Ingredients
–   2–4 tbsp raw apple
    cider vinegar (use
    2 tbsp for dry hair,
    4 for oily hair)
–   5 drops rosemary
    essential oil
–   3 drops clary sage
    essential oil
–   3 drops cedar oil
    (optional, great for hair
    growth)

Equipment
–   Jar with lid, or bottle
    pump dispenser,
    sterilised

Method

1–2. Pour all the ingredients into the jar or bottle and add 300ml
(10½fl oz/1¼ cups) water.

3. Seal with the lid and shake vigorously. Use within one week.

To use the rinse, apply it all over the hair, concentrating on the
scalp, and leave for three minutes. If you're in a rush one minute
will do!

Rinse with warm water.

Follow with a conditioning treatment or, depending on your hair
type, it may be possible to supplement your conditioner with
this rinse. Remember to shake the container again before each
subsequent use.

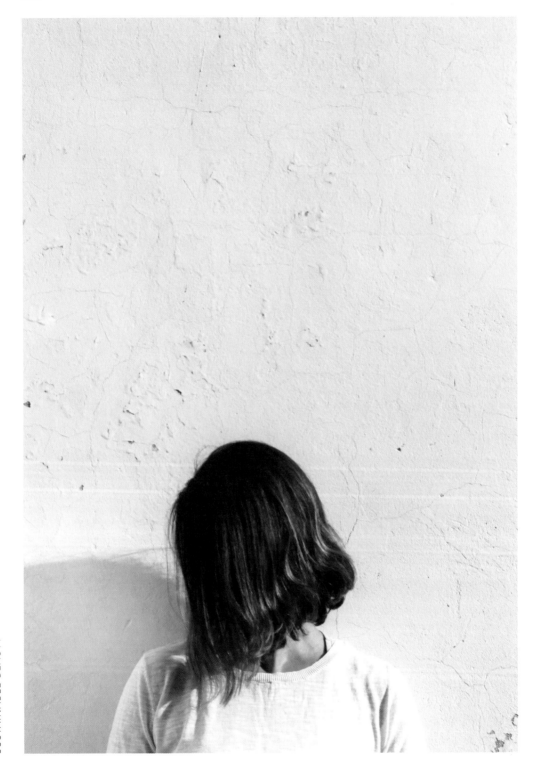

Ingredients to be aware of

Silicones

Silicones have been used in personal care products since the '50s. Initially limited to skincare items, their use has spread into hair-care products and treatments. Silicones used in hair-care give shine, smoothness and slip, making it easier to detangle hair and style. Natural shine is when the hair is properly hydrated and the cuticle is flat so light reflects off the hair. Silicone sticks to the hair creating a plastic-like film – think of it like a fake shine. It seals the hair shaft completely preventing moisture and nutrients from penetrating, so over time it will make hair lifeless, brittle and dull. Without regular treatment with a clarifying shampoo (shampoo with surfactants) to remove the silicones, it can lead to damage and breakage. It's like a hair merry-go-round because the clarifying shampoos are necessary to remove the silicones, but they are themselves drying. Look on labels for ingredients ending in 'cone', including dimethicone, methicone, amodimethicone, dimethiconol and cyclomethicone/cyclopentasiloxane.

Because of these issues, the beauty industry started to introduce water-soluble silicones which, you've guessed it, are much easier to remove. Apple cider vinegar (ACV) is a natural alternative to remove silicone build-up. My hair healing rinse (see page 101) is an ACV rinse that is simple to make and easy to use.

Propellants

Propellants are chemicals used to force fluid out of a can, so they are used in hairsprays, anti-perspirants and other aerosol products. In the '70s and '80s, propellants vinyl chloride and methylene chloride were used extensively in hairsprays. Both were eventually banned by the Food and Drug Administration (FDA) in the US due to their links to cancer. Hairspray manufacturers today advise that hairsprays should be used in a well-ventilated space, and are deemed safe. However, is there enough research to know if there are any long-term health impacts of using propellant sprays? It's something to think about when purchasing self-care products. Popular propellants in today's aerosol sprays include propane, butane, isobutane, carbon dioxide, nitrous oxide and dimethyl ether.

Surfactants

These ingredients are mainly added to products to remove excess sebum, dirt and oil from the hair. They also create foam and lather, neither of which are needed to actually clean the skin and hair. The only reason products are formulated with a foaming agent is for user experience. Heavy surfactants will be on the ingredients list as sodium laureth, myreth, lauryl sulphate, sodium coco sulphate and ammonium lauryl and laureth sulphate. Milder surfactants are sodium cocyl isethionate, cocamidopropyl betaine, sodium lauryl sulphoacetate and sodium lauryl glucose carboxylate. Naturally derived surfactants are much milder and gentler; they are better for your long-term hair health. Look out for coco glucoside, lauryl glucoside, sucrose cocoate, caprylyl/capryl glucoside and decyl glucoside. The latter created the most foam during an independent test, so if you feel you can't give up the foam, then look out for that ingredient.

Bedtime bliss and sweet sleep mists

Quality of sleep is a foundational element of our health, mind and general wellbeing. When our sleep patterns are disturbed, we witness a negative impact on every level of our lives. Here to help are my two tried-and-tested pillow mists. Bedtime bliss is a soothing, floral scent that aids relaxation and positive mood. The sweet, woody scent of the sweet sleep mist is great for grounding and encouraging a deep, replenishing sleep. All you need is five minutes and a clean bottle with an atomiser pump spray.

Ingredients

Bedtime bliss
- 30ml (1fl oz/2 tbsp) alcohol (try vodka or isopropyl, which is easy to buy online)
- 4 drops pure rose essential oil
- 3 drops lavender essential oil
- 3 drops roman chamomile essential oil
- 2 drops peppermint essential oil

Sweet sleep
- 30ml (1fl oz/2 tbsp) alcohol
- 8 drops vetiver essential oil
- 6 drops vervain essential oil
- 5 drops mandarin essential oil
- 4 drops lavender essential oil

Equipment
- Clean glass jar with lid
- Funnel
- Repurposed glass bottle with pump dispenser, sterilised

Method

1. Put the alcohol and essential oils in the jar, along with 30ml (1fl oz/2 tbsp) water.

2. Place the lid on the jar and shake vigorously.

3. Using the funnel, decant the liquid into the spray bottle and leave for 24 hours to infuse.

To use, spray a fine mist over your pillows and bedding. You might try a deep breathing technique, a mediation or a visualisation to further enhance your journey into dreamtime.

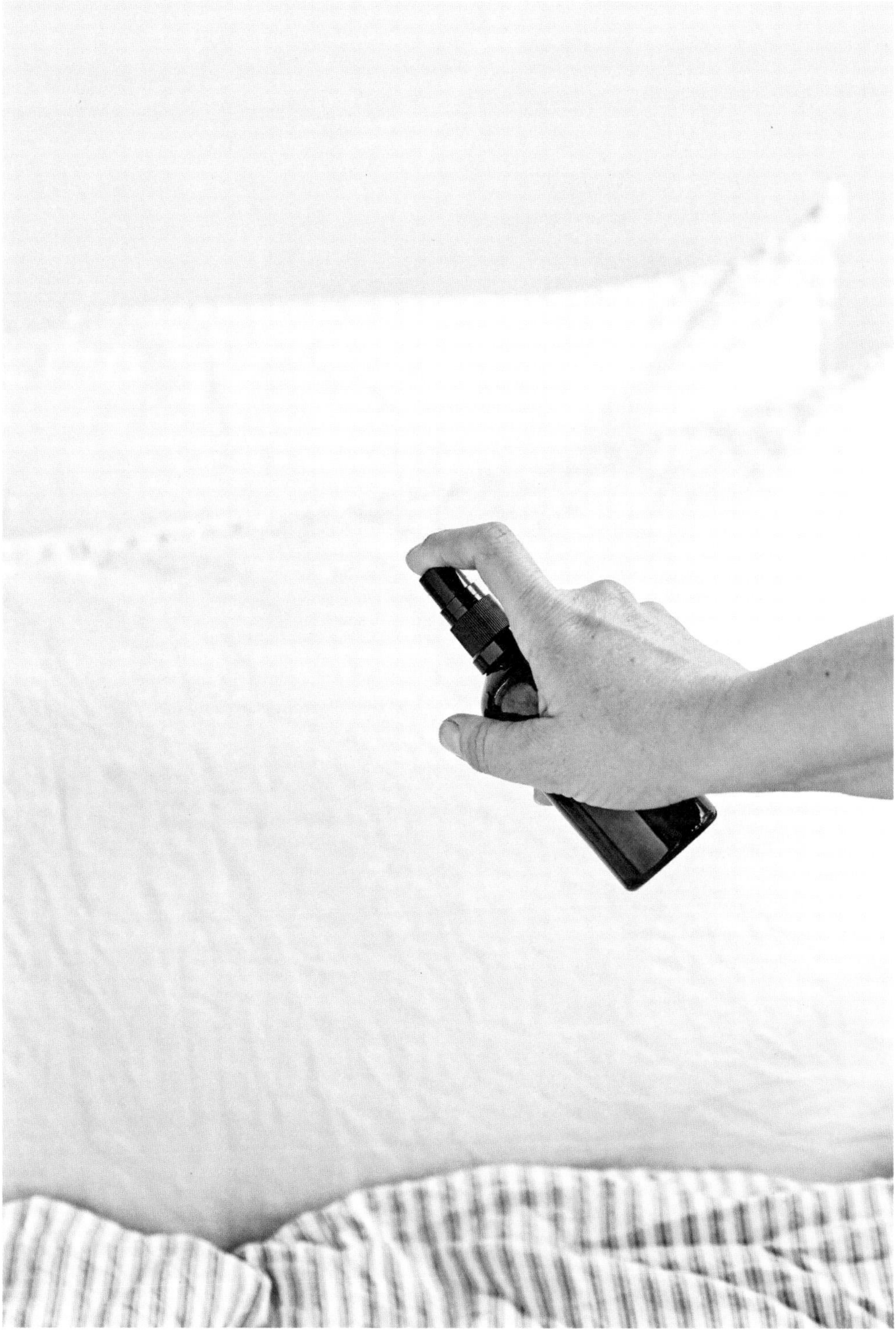

1

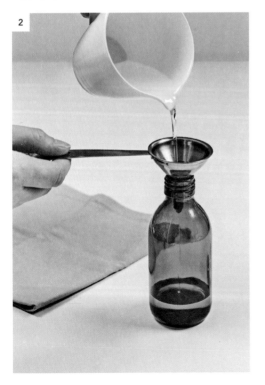

2

3

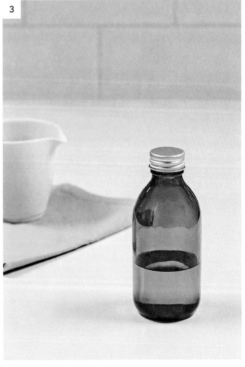

JJ's miracle moon oil for period pains

With just two ingredients, coconut (or almond) oil and clary sage essential oil, this is a tonic for the tumults of periods, which are often a source of pain and discomfort as well as headaches, nausea and so many other unpleasant symptoms each month. Clary sage has a spectrum of properties. Not only is it a phytoestrogen oil – it mimics oestrogen – but it is also anti-spasmodic (therefore soothing uterine contractions), tension reducing, anxiety calming, and it improves sleep quality. It works; I've been using my miracle moon oil for years.

Ingredients
– 64ml (2¼fl oz/¼ cup) fractionated (liquid) coconut oil (or almond oil)
– 4 drops clary sage essential oil
– 2 drops of either geranium or lavender essential oil (optional: day use)
– 2 drops lavender essential oil (optional: night use)

Equipment
– Small jug or cup
– Funnel
– Repurposed bottle or jar, sterilised

Method
1. In a cup or jug, mix together the coconut oil, clary sage essential oil, and any optional essential oils, if using.

2–3. Decant into a bottle or jar, using the funnel and store in a cool, dark place until needed.

To use, massage the tonic on dry skin – ideally after a bath and before bed – spending time calmly rubbing the oil onto your belly and lower back.

Spiced tooth powder

I don't recommend using this zingy tooth powder all the time, but it's an effective alternative to toothpaste several times a week. It's super easy to make, and you'll probably already have the ingredients lolloping around your kitchen: the baking soda is a mild abrasive, alkaline and assists in neutralising acid in the mouth; the salt is anti-bacterial, anti-microbial and a natural disinfectant; clove has anti-inflammatory properties (great for the gums), is anti-microbial, and has a local anaesthetic element which soothes sore teeth; finally, cinnamon is anti-bacterial, anti-viral, anti-fungal – all that and it adds a welcome sweetness to the mix.

Ingredients
– 5 tsp baking powder
  or bicarbonate of soda
  (baking soda)
– 2 tsp ground sea salt
  or Himalayan pink salt
  granules
– ½ tsp ground cloves
– 1 tsp ground cinnamon

Equipment
– Mixing bowl
– Wooden spoon
– Repurposed glass jar
  with lid, sterilised
– Toothbrush

Method
1. Add all the ingredients to the mixing bowl and mix together with the wooden spoon.

2. Decant into the jar, seal and store in a cool dark place until use.

When you want to glorify your gnashers, simply wet your toothbrush and then dip it into the jar and brush.

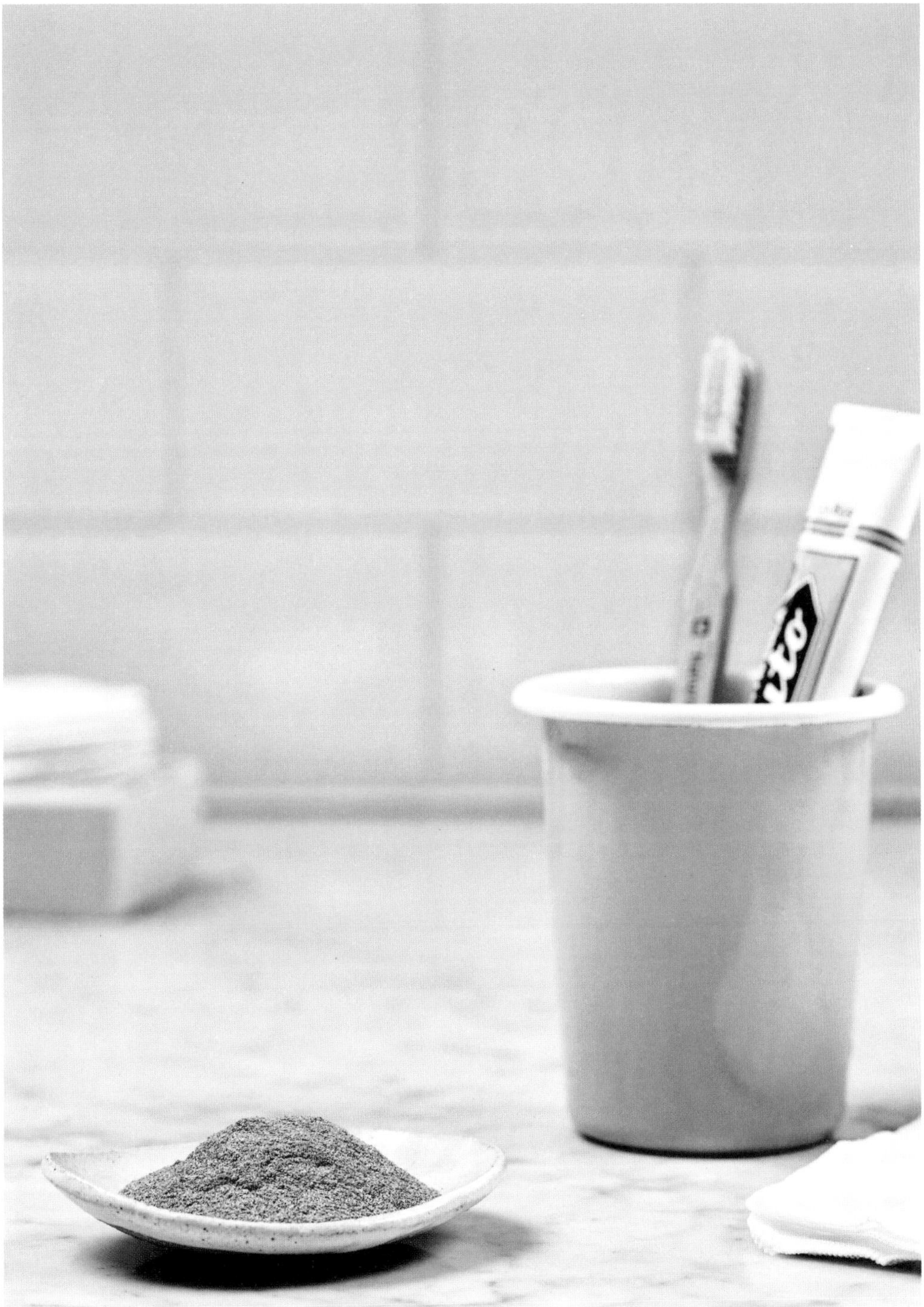

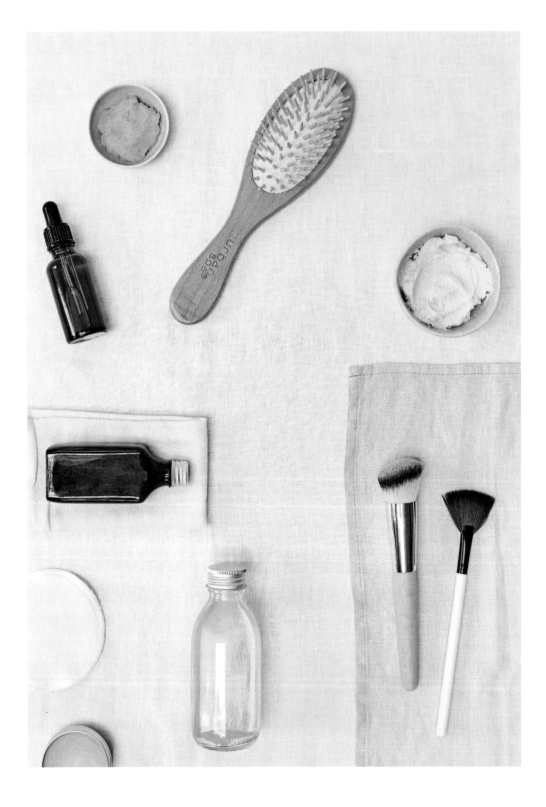

Mindful make-up

—

The beauty industry is full of trends, much like the fashion industry. It's designed to keep selling you product after product. Rather than following trends, discover what works for you. Learn to edit what you use, and incorporate slow beauty techniques for classic, natural beauty that will see you through your life. Like a capsule wardrobe, you can then use that base knowledge to introduce trend products, if you fancy. However, while it's fun to have the odd specialist product, if you want to reduce and simplify your make-up, be conscious of only investing in what you really need. Our over-consumption is having catastrophic effects on our planet, and our mental health too. If you have fewer, more carefully chosen products, everything has breathing space. You'll feel more organised, and the act of applying make-up becomes ritualised and joyful, rather than a rummage, a rush and a frenzy.

If your make-up bag is full of beautiful, edited products you cherish, you will use them until they're finished. Add extra items here and there, but stick to the basics, and you won't be swayed by spontaneous purchases that promise to change your life. These often never see the light of day and just create clutter.

Mindful make up and slow beauty are a philosophy. When we apply our beauty products, it's an opportunity to reconnect, be present and check in with ourselves. In a world where it's easy to get lost in a digital soup, even if it's just for a few minutes, your beauty and make-up routine offers time to really look at your face, touch your skin and understand in that moment, that you are creative. Don't do what you do every day just because you think you should. Make up is an art form and you are an artist. Is it a day when you need a bright lipstick, or nothing more than mascara and lip balm? Be conscious of how you feel and what you need. Apply your products in good lighting, clean your make up bag, cosmetics and brushes regularly so they are more enjoyable to use. Your carefully chosen beauty products enhance your visual image, which increases self esteem and confidence to face the outer world.

Start with products for a good base: a concealer, a foundation and a setting powder. For eyes, keep a versatile palette of matte and shimmer nude eyeshadows according to your skin tone. Within that palette should be a matte colour that can double up as a contour and also a colour to fill in your brows. The darker colours in the palette can be used wet as eyeliners, if you want to replace pencil or gel liners. Invest in a good black mascara, and don't bother with other colours unless you regularly use them. Bronzer adds warmth to your skin and can also be used as an eyeshadow. Blusher will add life to your complexion, but stick to one or two colours. Multi-use cream blushers can also be used on the lips, and lipsticks as cream blushers. I love highlighter but it's not essential if you take good care of your skin. Your nude eyeshadow palette can contain a colour you can double up as a highlighter. Add lip balm to it and it becomes a cream highlighter. Lip balm can also be used as a natural invisible highlighter and as a mixing medium with your lip colour to create a tinted balm. Have a day and evening lip colour, and add a lip pencil if you want more definition.

Really consider each product you buy. Look at the ingredients, ask yourself how you can use it as a multi-use product, find out where it is made, and what the packaging is made from. Be as conscious as you can about where your products go at the end of their life; read the Our Beautiful Planet chapter on pages 30–39 for how to dispose of them ethically.

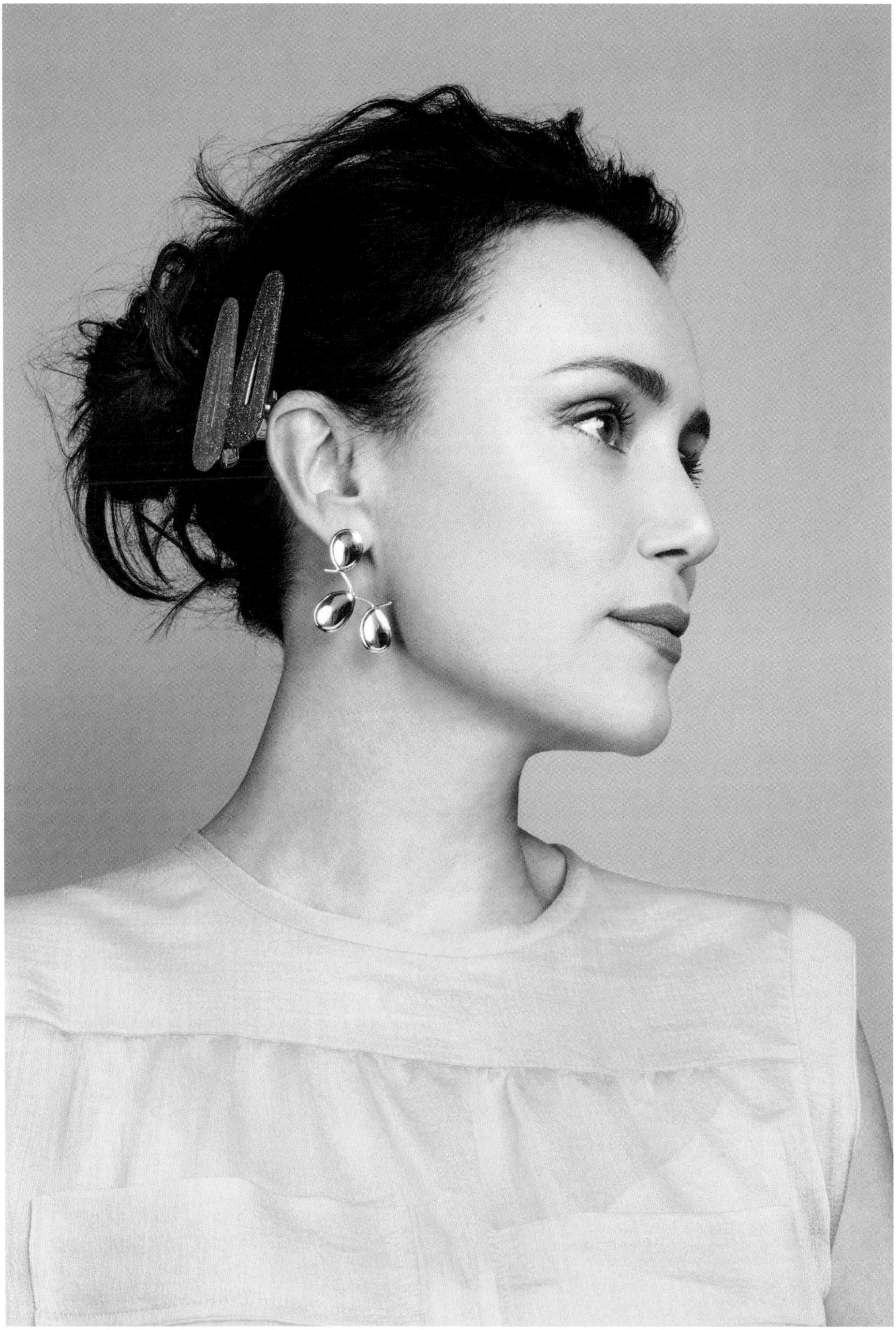

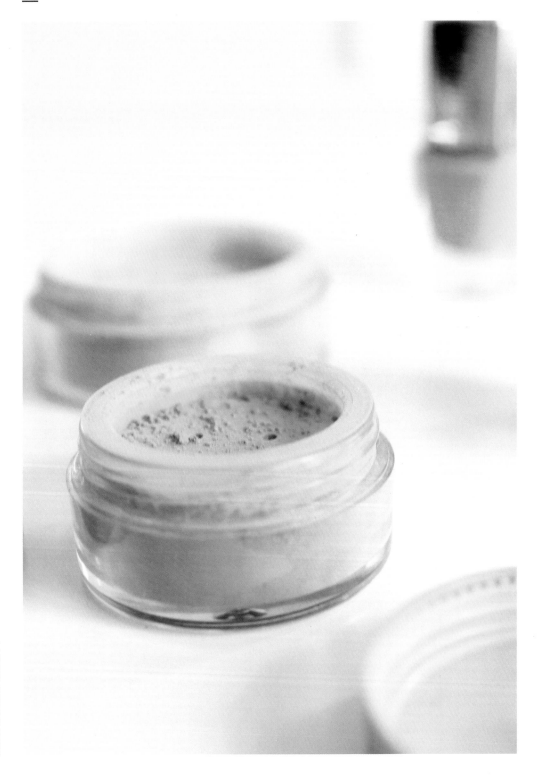

Face

—

Foundation, concealer and powder

Most people will use a foundation base in their beauty routine. Unless you are blessed with great skin and don't need it, or you just don't like the feel of it on your skin, a foundation is something I would definitely recommend. Even if you only wear a small amount, foundation makes the rest of your make-up look better. If you don't enjoy wearing make-up, a bit of base will even out your skin tone and generally make you look a little fresher. Bases come in many different forms: liquid, cream, powder, sheer, tinted moisturiser, beauty balm, CC cream, DD cream – all quite confusing really. Almost everyone will look great with a tinted moisturiser and concealer. They're the products I use most on my clients and myself, and they achieve the look that many of us are aiming for – a bit healthier, brighter and perkier. Your base can be finished with setting powder. I say 'can be' because it doesn't have to be. If you love an all-over radiance, don't powder; your base will look gorgeous and natural. If you want to, just apply it to the T-zone or even what I call the 'triangle zone' – the top section of the forehead, the sides of the nose and the entire top lip. The small area between the brows looks lovely with a bit of sheen. You can also use sustainable blotting papers instead of powder.

I often get asked whether to 'bake' foundation. This is an Instagram technique that involves placing as much powder over your foundation as you can, leaving it to 'bake' before brushing it away. If you love doing that, keep going and don't listen to me. However, if you've never done it, don't. You'll dry out your skin in a New York second. The foundation will make you look like Elizabeth I, and leave your skin feeling tight and dehydrated. Keep it for Instagram.

Liquid foundation
Moisturising, mattifying or any level in-between, there is a liquid foundation option out there for everyone. Full coverage matte foundations are popular, but if you want a natural look, avoid this type of formulation. They look good in front of a ring light on Instagram, but in natural daylight, appear heavy, chalky and ageing. If you want greater coverage, look for a thicker cream foundation that generally comes in pot form. This product will give full coverage but is less likely to look cakey and mask-like. Water-based foundations are the gentlest on the skin and will keep skin hydrated. They are great on days you want less coverage. Add a bit of moisturiser to any foundation to create a thinner consistency [1].

Pressed cream
Usually in compact or stick form, pressed creams are a great two-in-one product as it's also buildable as a concealer. Apply with a deft hand as too much cream foundation can look heavy. Creams mainly suit normal skin types. They are a great option for oily skins, and depending on the formulation, they also often suit dry skin. However, prep and moisturise the skin well beforehand, as they can highlight dry patches [2].

Sheer foundation
This product does what it says on the tin. A good option if you prefer a lightweight product on your skin. Suits all skin types [3].

Tinted moisturiser
For all skin types, especially mature skin, this is lighter in texture than a liquid foundation, with a luminous finish due to added hydrating skincare ingredients. A tinted moisturiser looks great on most people. It's a good option if you have dry skin or if you want radiance. Great for daytime or work and as your regular base. When you need more coverage, add concealer, where needed. A fantastic all-rounder [4].

BB (beauty balm)
Essentially turbo-charged tinted moisturisers, these are lightweight bases with added skin care benefits, often including SPF protection. Generally, they offer more coverage than a tinted moisturiser. Available for all skin types [5].

CC cream (colour correcting cream)
Supposedly lighter in texture than a BB cream, CC cream has clever colour-adapting pigments to reduce redness, discoloration and a sallow complexion [6].

DD cream (daily defence cream)
Basically BB creams with added anti-ageing and pollution-protecting ingredients. Designed to target fine lines and wrinkles, they work well with mature skins [7].

Powder foundation
A two-in-one foundation and powder, used lightly, these foundations make a good multi-use product, but when applied too heavily, they will look chalky. Avoid at all costs if you have dry skin, or are over 30 [8].

Mineral powder foundations
Formulated from crushed minerals, these foundations can be a great option for most skin types. However, be wary of any containing bismuth oxychloride. It's an irritating little bugger of an ingredient found in some mineral powders, so steer clear of those brands if you have sensitive skin. Some mineral powder foundations can give a silvered finish due to their use of mica. Apply these lightly, or else you could end up looking like the Tin Man from *The Wizard of Oz*. If you have very dry and/or mature skin, I would avoid any powder foundation unless it's a lightweight texture [9].

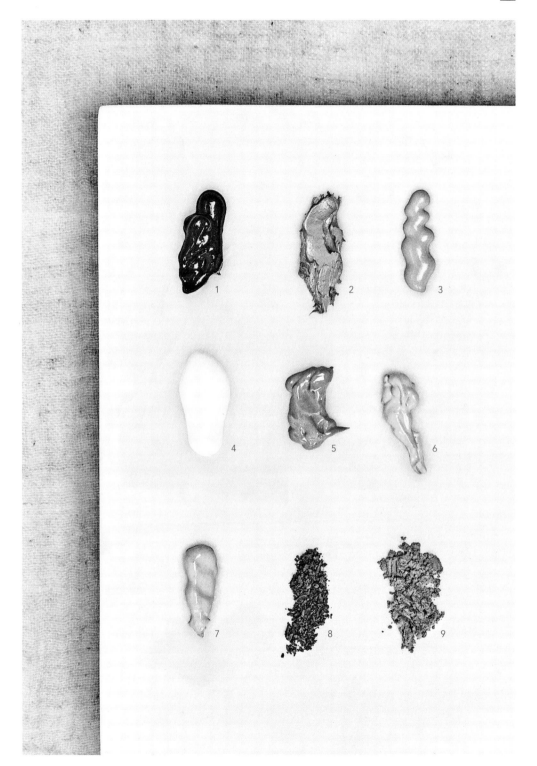

Application techniques

Tinted moisturisers, BB, CC, DD creams and sheer foundations apply and blend really well using your fingers, which is also a very sustainable way to apply product. Liquid foundations and cream foundations have several ways you can apply and blend them: fingers, foundation brushes, flat-topped kabuki brushes, sponges and beauty blenders. There are a lot of options. From a sustainable point of view, clean fingers and well-made brushes are a better option than sponges and beauty blenders, although the latter will work well for people with motor difficulties. Powder and mineral foundations are best applied with a medium-sized powder brush. Many mineral foundations require a buffing application technique. Place the brush into the powder, tap off the excess and buff onto the skin in circular motions. Make sure the brush you use is the right size. If it's too big, you won't be able to buff properly, and if it's too small, you'll be there all day.

BEAUTY DILEMMA: How do you find the right colour for you?

How do you find the right colour for you?
Stripe your selected range of foundation colours just above your jawline. Check in a mirror in daylight. The colour that 'disappears' is your foundation. If you have different tones of skin on different parts of your face, use the same stripe method on the relevant areas in order to find the right colour.

Concealers

A concealer is a useful skin product for hiding blemishes, dark circles and areas of discoloration, such as around the nose. An under eye concealer is thinner in consistency, so more adaptable to the fine skin in that area of your face. Under eye concealers often have added illuminating ingredients, so can be useful as a highlighter. If you have a cream highlighter and want to use it for under eyes, just add a bit of serum or moisturiser to sheer out the texture.

TECHNIQUE: For liquid under-eye concealer, apply straight from the applicator. Dot along the orbital bone from the inner corner to about three quarters of the way across. Using your ring finger, gently pat the product until it's fully blended. Don't forget the inner corner – apply and blend right up to the brow bone. This area is naturally shadowed by your nose, so lifting this section of your face will instantly brighten your eyes. Cream concealer can be placed on the back of your hand using a spatula, then warm with your ring finger and apply directly to the area. Any concealer application will benefit from using a soft brush to blend and blur the edges. I also love to use foundation or concealer if I've applied too much cream blusher. Apply over the whole blush area if the colour is too deep, or just around the edges if there are obvious lines.

BEAUTY DILEMMA: If you have lots of spots or acne, should you use a full coverage foundation and heavy concealer?

If you have lots of spots or acne, should you use a full coverage foundation and heavy concealer? No. You can still achieve a natural-looking skin just by taking a bit more time and care with your base. Try to look beyond your spots at your skin. Match it to a relevant base like a tinted moisturiser, then spend some time concealing your spots individually, rather than masking over your whole skin. That is a quicker technique of course, but you'll get a more beautiful base with this slow beauty technique.

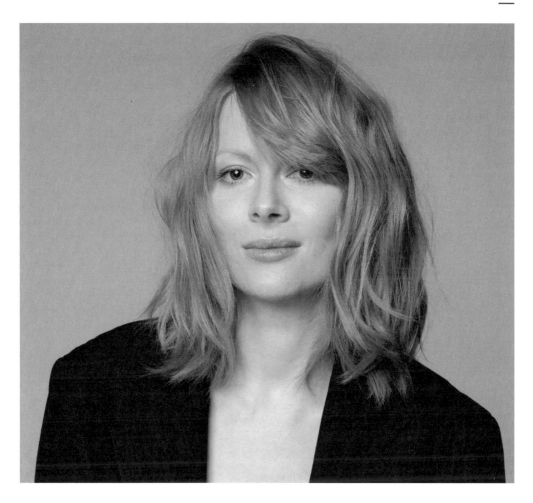

Setting powder ·

This is a fine colourless powder (translucent) used to take off any shine from the face and enhance the longevity of your make-up. It comes loose or in a pressed compact. The latter is more useful for touch-ups throughout the day, however it tends to come in a mirrored compact that is not recyclable curbside. Compacts have to be sent off for specialist recycling or sadly thrown in your rubbish. Many loose powders come in plastic containers that can generally be recycled in your recycling bin.

TECHNIQUE: I personally favour small powder brushes over large brushes or powder puffs to apply, as you can be more specific with where you place powder. Soft brushes pick up less product than a dense brush and are a better option for slowly layering on product. If you take your time, powdering this way keeps your look natural and you won't over-powder. Pick up the powder on your brush and tap off excess before applying to your skin. Keep slowly adding powder and buffing into the skin until you are happy with the result.

Contour and highlight

Contouring has become a massive part of the beauty industry in the last few years. It was always a simple technique to create more defined cheekbones, a sharper jawline and, perhaps, a thinner nose. Instagram has been big in promoting a plethora of contouring products, from powders to creams to whole palettes. However, Instagram is fun, but it's not reality. It does not reflect how everyone should apply make-up. Think of those full-on technique placements of contour and highlight as theatre, and the make-up like theatre make-up. Would you honestly want to go to the local shop wearing theatre make-up?

Not everyone suits contouring. Those with a naturally thinner face do not need it, neither does anyone whose facial shape has thinned through age. This is because contouring gives the illusion of slimming and defining, and so only use it if that is what you want. Think of contouring as shadow, so where you want definition or shape, that's where you apply contour. A mistake many people make is that they bring their cheek contour down too far towards their mouth. If you bring it beyond your actual cheekbone, you will create a drawn look to your face, rather than a healthy one. Remember, you always want to lift up with make-up, not drag down. Stick to simple techniques and you can't go wrong.

Contouring powder

This is the easiest texture to apply and the most popular contouring product. Choose a powder with minimum shimmer and a cooler tone. Personally, I don't like any contour colours that have warmth, no matter what skin tone you are. Warmth is for bronzer. A matte texture creates a more successful contour with the least amount of product. I can't say it enough, but for a natural look, subtlety and blending is the key.

TECHNIQUE: Use a small to medium-sized powder brush, angled, flat or round. Place in the powder and tap off the excess. Start underneath the cheekbone close to your ear and sweep the contour along the edge of your cheekbone. Use small sweeps flicking up and along to blend in, and a clean soft brush to buff any obvious edges. Do not place contour beyond your cheekbone. Stop at the edge of your bone, before it starts to round. You are creating more definition but you want to still have lift in your face. To slim the top part of your face, use circular movements over your temples, then go along the hairline across your forehead with what's left on the brush. For jawline definition, place the brush on the underside of the jaw, remembering to take the contour right up to the ear. Regarding the nose area, take a small soft eyeshadow brush and gently sweep down the sides of the nose. Any contouring on the nose can look really obvious, so go lightly. Alternatively, create a highlight vertically down the bridge of your nose; this gives the illusion of thinning without the need for contour.

Contour cream

This comes in compact, palette or stick form. Creams go on top of creams, so apply over a liquid or cream base or moisturised skin. Contour creams can multi-use as a cream eyeshadow, applied lightly to avoid creasing.

TECHNIQUE: The key to contour cream application is the brush. Use a small flat foundation brush or a medium-sized angled brush. Apply to the same areas as you would with contour powder, blending with a soft buffing brush, sponge or fingers. If you want to powder over, it's best to do this once all cream products have been applied, including base, contour, blush and highlight.

TECHNIQUE: Powders, creams and liquid highlighters can be applied to both face and body, using brushes, fingers and sponges. Colour-wise, look to your skin tone: pale skins suit oyster, champagne, apricot and pink tones, while olive and medium to darker skin tones suit bronze and golden highlights.

Apply on areas such as the top of cheekbones, bridge of the nose, above the brow arch, on the brow bone, centre of the forehead, chin and cupid's bow. I also like to press a finger of highlighter onto the tip of the nose, inner corner of the eyes, eyelids and between the eyebrows. I don't personally like anything more than a hint of glow on the brow bone and forehead, as I like to keep highlights there subtle. Body-wise, apply to the collar bone, shoulders and down the

centre of the shins (apparently this makes legs look longer). You don't, of course, need to apply highlighter to all these areas, only where you want a glow. Visualise how healthy fresh skin looks, and how the light naturally bounces off it. This is what you can recreate with highlight.

I prefer a natural-looking glow, so I would advise against over-applying highlighter to where sweat glands are, namely the part of your cheeks nearest your nose, as you will just look sweaty. If you are a make-up artist getting a client ready for a red carpet look, or someone who wants to look good on camera, test out your highlighting products for flashback. This is the over reflective effect that flash photography can have on a highlighter.

Highlighting

Who doesn't want radiant skin lit by soft candlelight? If you haven't got it, fake it. Used subtly, highlighting will make you look brighter, refreshed, elevated, glowing, chic and downright gorgeous. Overuse it and you could be mistaken for actress Margaret Nolan in the James Bond classic, Goldfinger. Strobing is the name that's been given to using highlighting without contour. It basically involves highlighting areas of the face that light naturally hits, giving the illusion of light and shadow on the face without having to apply contour. Don't worry if it all sounds confusing – again, these are just terms that have been created to sell you products in a different way. Be careful of using highlighting products that are so full of shimmer and glitter that it distracts from the rest of your make-up. Avoid these products unless you want what I call 'mirror highlighting'.

Powder highlighters

These come in different strengths, from a light glow to full-on Pearly Queen. In my opinion, they are the easiest formulation to use, blending seamlessly over powdered skin, and are great for all ages and skin types. On days when you

look and feel tired, if you only do one thing, use powder highlighter on the inner corner of the eyes plus a coat of mascara. You'll instantly look brighter and fresher.

TECHNIQUE: Use a really soft brush. Soft fibres pick up less product and allow you to gradually layer the highlighter to your required luminosity. I like to use a fan brush on the cheekbones and a small soft brush for other areas of the face and body. Place the product on the brush and tap off any excess. Apply a small amount at first, blend, then take a step back and look in the mirror before deciding to apply more. Layering your product slowly will help you create a radiant glow exactly where you want it. If you do apply too much, use a clean brush to remove what you can, dab over the area with a tissue or powder puff, and dust lightly with translucent powder.

Liquid highlighter

Apply over or under your base on un-powdered skin. If you have an uneven skin texture, avoid them and stick to highlighter powders. Liquid highlighters come in varying strengths and some are highly pigmented, so if you are looking for full-on highlight, this is the formulation for you. Go easy if you prefer a more natural look, these shimmery liquids can be quite intense. If you like the texture of a liquid but want to reduce its flashy power, you can add a little into your foundation before applying, or apply separately under your foundation to blur the strength. If you are interested in make-up alchemy, they blend well with all other liquid formulations, such as foundation, liquid blusher and moisturiser, so you can formulate your own bespoke product. With liquids you get the most localised application, as opposed to a powder, which creates a more diffused highlight.

TECHNIQUE: Dot on the areas you want to highlight. You can use your finger, but I prefer a brush with liquids to fully blend in any edges. A beauty blender or sponge will be useful for anyone with motor difficulties.

Cream highlighter

Cream is my favourite formulation. These are available in compact, stick or palette form and are great for dry skin types. Cream highlighter can have added shimmer or can simply be a matt cream that is a couple of shades lighter than your skin tone. Matt textures work well with oily skin types who should avoid too much shimmer.

TECHNIQUE: Apply cream highlighter over your un-powdered base, or directly onto clean skin if you do not want to use a foundation. Pat onto the areas you wish to highlight with your middle finger and blend. This is my preferred method of application for creams, but you can also use brushes. I find sponges not precise enough for highlighting. If you are using a setting powder, this should be your last step. However, if you need to apply cream over powder, use a very light touch, else you'll disturb the make-up underneath. Experiment by mixing your cream highlighter with cream blusher for a beautiful, flushed radiance to the skin.

Invisible highlighter

What I'm referring to here is a clear product to reflect light, such as a balm or oil. You can apply it over a base, or straight onto clean skin for a very natural glow. Do not powder over this type of highlight as it can make the powder clump and stick. More suited to regular or dry skin types, the beauty of invisible highlighter is that there's no colour, just glow. The balm or oil will nourish your skin, which in turn will look amazing. I also use a serum concealer for invisible highlight, one that has sheen. If you have any pigmentation, this is a great way to add coverage and glow simultaneously. You are likely to have one or more of these products already in your bathroom cabinet or make-up bag, so invisible highlighting is a great way to sustainably swap out a separate highlighting product altogether!

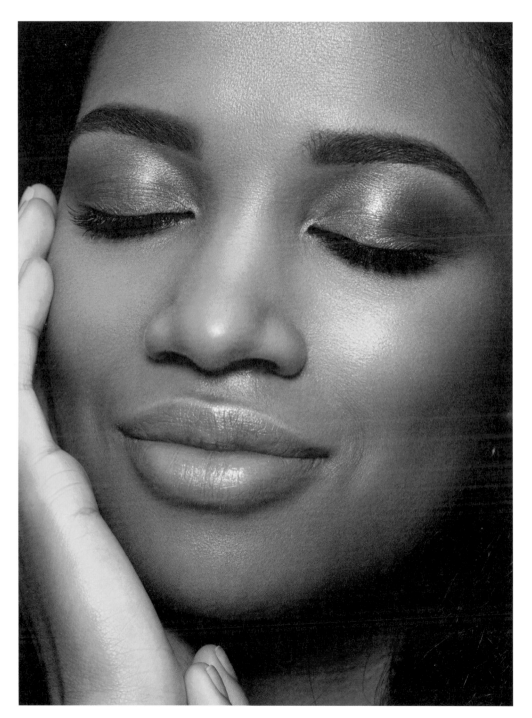

Blusher and bronzer

Blusher is everyone's best friend because it brightens dull skin instantly. Blush products come in many forms – powder, cream, liquid, balm, stick and gel. You don't need all of them, just one or two that work with your skin type and give you an immediate bloom. Bronzer is available in powder, cream, liquid and gel textures and lifts the entire skin tone by a shade or two. It's useful as an overall complexion enhancer, whereas blusher is placed more precisely. Blusher for me, is the product that brings your entire make-up look together. It links your eye make-up with your lip colour, however subtly it's applied. Both products are great multitaskers, and very useful to have in your mindful make-up bag. Bronzer can double up as a blusher, contour and eyeshadow.

Blusher can be used on the lips, even a powder formulation. Scrape off a small amount of your powder blush, mix in some lip balm and, voila, you have lipstick!

What blusher is right for you?

In terms of colour, there are no rules with blusher. Well, not any that I stick to! The only instance where you should be mindful of your blusher colour is if you have redness or rosacea. The best colours to minimise redness would be those with a tawny, bronze or peach undertone. Avoid pinks and reds. Texture-wise, think about your skin type: if you have oilier skin, you'll be best suited to a powder, and if you have dry skin, a cream formulation will counteract any dullness.

TECHNIQUE: With both bronzer and blusher (and highlighter), there is a guideline for choosing which texture to use. Cream on cream and powder on powder. For the simple reason it makes application easier and the products blend seamlessly. Therefore a powder blush or bronzer will be much easier to apply and blend over an already-powdered base, and a cream, liquid or gel product will blend better over an un-powdered base.

Bronzer is best placed around the edges of the face, under the cheekbones and along the jawline before blending in towards the centre of the face. A subtle amount can be added to the bridge of the nose and the chin, all the areas where the sun naturally tints the face. Powder bronzer is the easiest to apply with a big soft brush for all over diffused colour. Cream, liquid and gel bronzers are best applied with a foundation brush, a flat topped foundation brush or a sponge. For more specific placement, use fingers or a small foundation brush. Keep a clean brush to hand for buffing and blending. If you want a healthy glow without make-up, apply a pea-size amount of gel bronzer all over moisturized skin. Liquid bronzers can also be mixed in directly with your foundation.

When it comes to blusher, it's the same as highlighter, gradually layering is the best method to prevent you applying too much in one go. In terms of product placement, I find blush on the apple suits just about everyone. This is where you flush when you've been exercising or when you find someone attractive. Blusher placed here gives a fresh, plump, natural appearance and blusher on the cheekbones gives a more structured look.

Smile, find your 'apple' (the mound of your cheek) apply your product in the centre, blend outwards and slightly inwards. Alternatively, place your blusher along your cheekbone and blend. You want to eliminate any hard lines so buff lightly with a clean soft brush to blend any edges. Do not apply blush too far in towards the nose or you'll look like you are having a hot flush. It can work for a fashion shoot, but not for real life. Use the centre of your iris as the limit, or measure two fingers in from the side of your nose – your blusher shouldn't creep in further than that. Do not apply too far up toward the eye, otherwise your blush can look like a bruise. For those with motor challenges, a beauty blender sponge used with a cream blusher makes for an easier application.

BEAUTY DILEMMA: What to do if you apply too much blusher.

What to do if you apply too much blusher.

We've all gone in a bit heavy-handed with the blush, only to realise we look more like Coco the Clown than Coco Chanel. If you overdo it, there are a few things you can do to alleviate the situation. With powder blusher, you can blot off with a tissue or soft cloth, then dust over with some setting powder. If you have really overdone the colour, going over the area with a powder foundation will knock the colour right back. With a cream, liquid or gel, simply apply a little of your foundation over your blush. Use the foundation remnants on the brush or sponge that you first applied your foundation with.

Powder blusher

The most common type of blusher, which suits all skin types. Powders come in different finishes, from matte right through to full-on shimmer. Opt for a slight sheen rather than shimmer to give radiance which makes skin look healthy. Shimmer finish can draw attention to any bumps and large open pores. A matte texture, on the other hand, will diffuse those issues, and is generally the best option for oily skin.

TECHNIQUE: Powder blusher is best applied slowly, with a light hand. I like using a fan brush as it only picks up a small amount of product each time, allowing you to build up colour easily. Small powder brushes are also very useful for more specific placement, and a soft buffer brush blends any edges. Always tap off the excess from your brush to avoid applying too much product.

Cream or gel blusher

I love cream and gel blush. Applied correctly, they give skin that lit-from-within glow that we all hanker after. You'll find gel blushers in tube or stick form, and creams in a pot, compact, tube or stick. They are ideal for dry and mature skin as they reflect light, adding radiance to the skin.

Liquid blusher

Liquids usually come in a glass or plastic container with an applicator. As with cream blush, use over unpowdered skin. The thin texture of liquid blush looks more like a second skin, so it's a good option if you want a light flush of colour and a crisp natural look.

TECHNIQUE: Apply either over foundation or on clean moisturized skin. You need to work quickly with liquid blush as it tends to set, which gives it longevity. Place it on the back your hand before applying so you have greater control. It's important to start with a really small amount and build up, as a little goes a very long way. As with cream and gel blush, place a little on the apple of your cheek or your cheekbones. Take your middle finger or a foundation brush and start to blend, adding more product where needed. Blend away any obvious edges with a little foundation.

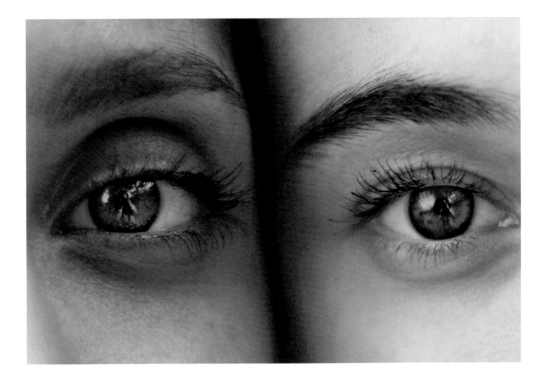

Eyes

—

Would you like to wear eye make-up but don't know how? It's an area of make-up that confuses people to the extent that they don't wear it at all. Learning some easy, quick application methods can change that habit and make all the difference to how you feel when you walk out the door. Make-up can help increase our self-esteem because when we think that we look our best, we feel good. In effect, it's an act of self-care and self-expression.

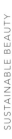

Brows

I love more than anything, a natural brow that has never been plucked, waxed, threaded, tattooed, microbladed, laminated or shaved. It has a genetically good shape and is full and vibrant. Those brows are like a rare species of bird; you only see them on a few occasions in your lifetime. Most of us have attacked our brows at some point in our life, and have learnt the hard way that brow hair doesn't always grow back. Permanent make up is one of many brow treatments now available, but a word of caution before you sign up. Be absolutely sure this is the right treatment for you, and be sure of the shape you want before you commit. Trends come and go, but permanent make up doesn't!

Filling in the natural brow

Once you've got the natural shape you want, you can use products to enhance your brows. Over-plucking or the ageing process can create gaps that do look better filled in if you want to look groomed. Pencils, stencils, shadows, pomades, coloured waxes, markers, mascaras, the list goes on. The perfect colour to fill your brows will match your brow colour, not your hair colour. Brows tend to be a slightly cooler tone than your hair; I like to go a shade or two lighter with brow product so they are not over defined and do not dominate your face. Even if you have warm tones in your hair, cool tones work better for brows. Just think flat colours with a bit of grey in them: ash for blonde and light brown hair, charcoal for brunettes; and grey suits just about everyone. Red hair is a little different and you can use slightly warm tones. Ginger hair and strawberry blondes look good with an ashy blonde, light grey taupe or a warm blonde tone. If you are a darker ginger or auburn brunette, then a flat cool brown tone or a light warm brown tone work well. Grey hair suits a light or dark grey taupe, or grey, and if you have black hair, you lucky thing, you can wear matching black brow products.

TECHNIQUE: If you want to pluck your brows, this is an old-school brow-plucking guide, which most make-up artists advocate. Give your brows a quick brush through in the direction you like them. Place a thin make-up brush or tail comb up against the side of your nose and straight up towards your brow. Any brow hair that sits over the line on the inner edge can be removed. The same applies to the outer corner of your brow. Place the brush/comb diagonally on the edge of your nostril, lining it up with the outer corner of your eye. The handle of the tail comb or make-up brush will sit on your brow. Any brow hair beyond that line can be removed. When it comes to altering the shape of your brows proceed with caution. If in doubt, take a pencil the same colour as your skin tone and draw over the hairs you are considering removing. Take a step back and look in a mirror. Does it look good, or will it create an odd shape? If you are happy, tweeze them out. You'll save yourself time and frustration if you choose a sharp, slanted tweezer from a reputable brand. Good tools and a gentle stretch of the skin will achieve removal with the least amount of pain. Expect the odd sneeze – the pain of plucking can cause a fake sneeze signal in nearby nerve endings. Rubbing ice over the area before plucking, will reduce inflammation and redness. If you've grabbed the tweezers, attempted a brow shape and it hasn't worked as you'd hoped, don't fret. Pure castor oil is a great way of naturally stimulating brow growth. Use a spoolie brush (eyebrow brush), or an old mascara wand to apply it, as the combing action stimulates hair growth.

MINDFUL MAKE-UP

MY TOP 15 NATURAL BROWS

- Singer-songwriter Solange Knowles
- Actress Brooke Shields
- Model Charli Howard
- Model Natalia Castellar Calvani
- Actress Zendaya
- Actress Amandla Stenberg
- Actress Mollie Windsor
- Actress Aisling Bea

- Actress Florence Pugh
- Actress Lily Newmark
- Actress Millie Brady
- Actress Jessie Barden
- Actress Hayley Squires
- Actress Jodie Comer
- Actress Lily Collins

TECHNIQUE: Stick to a pencil or shadow for light filling and a pomade for deeper filling. Brush through your brows with an old mascara wand or a spoolie brush, and if necessary, apply a lightweight gel, soap, clear balm or wax to keep hairs in place. Direction-wise, brush upwards first, then brush outwards with a slight angle for a natural shape. I favour angled or microfine pencil products, and if using a powder or pomade, dab an angled brush into your product, then tap on the back of your hand to remove excess. My favourite-ever brow product was an eyeshadow; it was just the perfect colour, so try one of your eyeshadows and sustainably swap out a separate brow product. My preference is a natural brow shape as opposed to a harsher squared off brow. Therefore, I always fill the inner corner last so there is the least amount of product on the brush. One technique I like to use is by drawing a soft horizontal line under the inner corner of the brow. Then use a spoolie brow brush to blend the product upwards through the brow leaving just a faint line. This gives what I call a base line, and makes it easier to apply further upward strokes, as you have that starting guideline in place.

There are times when this, and a brush through, is the only thing I do to the brow.

You don't need to load your entire brow with product. If you fill the gaps first, stand back and observe, then you can make a call as to whether you need more. Keep brush and pencil strokes weightless. Control the pressure by resting your elbow on a flat surface and/or support your wrist with your other hand. You might find it easier to lean over and look downwards into a mirror placed flat on a table, so you can rest your whole forearm on the surface. Don't press too hard on the brow and you should be able to maintain light, feathery strokes. If you do apply more product than you'd intended, just run a spoolie brush through your brows, which will knock back the intensity and blend in the colour. Keep looking in the mirror to check your work until you are happy with the result. When grooming your other brow, remember the saying 'sisters not twins'. Nobody's brows are totally symmetrical, so don't stress about them looking exactly the same. Enjoy their individuality.

SUSTAINABLE BEAUTY

Eye make-up

Concealer

Many of us have dark circles we'd like to cover. We have them for many reasons, some we can change – for example, drinking enough water, and getting enough sleep – and some we can't, like genetics. However, we can all work some magic with a bit of concealer. Serum-style concealers are lightweight but highly pigmented. You get good coverage, and the formulation doesn't cake around the eyes. I use these concealers anywhere on the face. A concealer in a pot is likely to have more sustainable packaging, as applicators in tubes tend to be non-recyclable. If the texture of your concealer is too heavy for the eye area, mix in some skincare serum or moisturiser, in order to create a thinner consistency (check that your skincare products can be used around the eye first). If you have loose skin and deeper wrinkles under the eye area, stretch the skin gently to flatten out wrinkles before you apply. I don't normally advise stretching the eye area, but you need to press the product into the wrinkles, otherwise it will sit on top of the skin giving the illusion of deeper wrinkles. Alternatively, opt for a more illuminating under-eye product, as they generally have a thinner consistency, so work well with mature skin. The illuminating particles bounce light off the dark shadow rather than cover it, but the thinner consistency won't sit on top of any wrinkles. If you have lines on the outer corner of the eye, apply concealer, starting from the inner corner and finishing at three-quarters of the way along the under-eye area. Blend with your ring finger or a soft brush. Don't forget the inner corner recess of the eye. It's easily passed over as we concentrate on underneath the eye, but concealer placed there can work wonders at brightening and lifting. To set the concealer, use the finest powder you can find. This will knock back any shine and the fine texture won't make your under-eyes look dry. Keeping the shine can also be beneficial by reflecting light off the area, à la Gillian Anderson, so you don't have to.

THE BENEFITS:

Hygiene – you're using a separate brush to apply, which you don't place back in the tube. The brush can easily be washed after each application.

Length of use – tube mascaras need to be replaced every three or four months, due to bacteria build-up, whereas cake mascaras can last up to two years. Not that it will ever last that long, if, like me, you love mascara.

Control – you can't control how much product comes out on the brush of regular mascaras, whereas with cake you can. If one day you want less product for a more natural look, it's easy!

Ingredients – a low ingredient count means they are better for sensitive eyes.

Other uses – have dark hair and need a root touch up? No problem: just use your cake mascara.

Sustainability – if all that wasn't enough to convince you, cake mascaras usually come in a recyclable refillable tin. You can buy a refill when you've finished, recycle it or repurpose the tin to hold safety pins, bobby pins etc.

Mascara – and the case for cake mascara

Make a sustainable swap to cake mascara. There are not many brands that offer them, but hunt around and you can find them. They are becoming more and more popular as people realise they can't recycle tube mascaras, so I expect to see more new releases. Use them with eyelash curlers if you want more lash lift.

Tube mascaras are a clever design, but so bad for the environment. Before their invention, cake mascaras were all people used. I say bring back the cake!

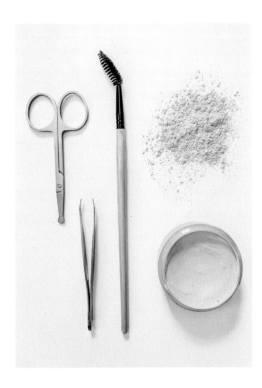

Eyeshadow

Unfortunately, most palettes are made with magnets – to hold in the shadows and to help keep the palette closed, therefore they are non-recyclable. When you purchase a ready-made palette, there will always be colours that you don't use as much, or not at all, so it's more sustainable to create your own palette of colours you will enjoy. You can purchase empty palettes quite easily and fill them with single eyeshadows – or add in a mix of blusher, bronzer and powder. Many brands now sell their products in individual refill format. Palettes made from recyclable materials such as card or sustainable bamboo are better options. Avoid magnets if possible, but if you can't, at least your refillable palette will last a lot longer.

TECHNIQUE: The technique is the same for both tube and cake mascara. As with eyeliner application, look down in a mirror. This allows you to really get to the roots of your lashes with both eyes open. A magnifying mirror is even better. Start at the roots and wiggle the brush to offload product. Then sweep the brush through your lashes. Use the tip of the brush to get the hard-to-reach lashes on the inner corner of the upper lash line. Covering those particular lashes will make your eyes look extra fluttery. I also like to use the tip for the lower lash line, sweeping back and forth or picking out individual lashes. However many coats you apply (I use one or two), put an extra coat on the upper outer lashes to wing them out and give extra definition. If there are any clumpy bits, just run your ring finger through your lashes, roots to tip and side to side, or press the clump between two fingers. This does the trick.

ESSENTIAL EYE KIT

If you are unsure what you actually need in your eye make-up kit, here is my list of essentials. Where relevant I've suggested the easiest-to-recycle packaging options.

- Concealer (glass pot)
- Cake mascara (black)
- Nude eyeshadow palette (buy refills and fill your own palette)
- Cream-coloured eyeliner (only if you suffer with red eyes)
- Black and brown eye pencil (crayon/pencil/gel)
- Spoolie brush for mascara application and brow grooming
- Angled brush for filling in brows with eyeshadow.

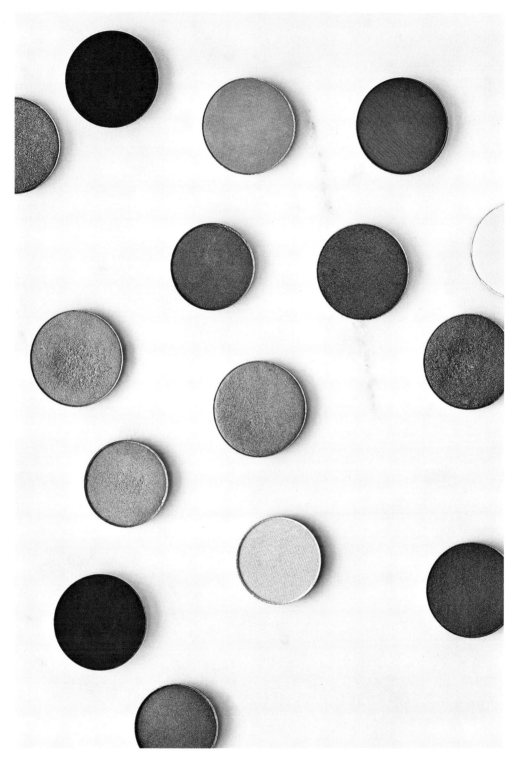

Eye make-up techniques

A natural eye

Simple natural eye make-up suits everyone. This technique is based on a wash of one colour around the eyes to frame them and give them enough definition, but in a natural way. It's so simple and chic, you can wear it anywhere and with anything. The trick is choosing the right eyeshadow tone. You are looking for one that is a similar colour to the natural skin tone of your eyelids, but a couple of shades darker. I prefer cooler tones for this look – cool taupes, mid flat browns, dark flat charcoal browns, purple, dark cool creams, dusky mauves, rose and grey pinks.

TECHNIQUE: Taking a small- to medium-sized eyeshadow brush, start applying the colour on the lids from lash to socket line, and use a smaller smudge brush to apply along the lower lash line. Then buff and blend with a clean, soft brush, using back-and-forth and small circular movements until the shadow has blended just above the socket line when you look straight ahead. Blend in the lower lash line with a smaller buffing brush so there are no harsh lines. With clean hands, dab your ring finger in an eye shadow lighter than your skin colour and gently press it in the inner corner of the eye. We tend to be darker in this area so this added brightness gives the eye a nice lift. Apply mascara and brush and fill brows. If you are tired and your eyes look a little red, take a cream pencil and apply to the waterline. I find white looks too harsh. Cream removes redness but still looks natural.

Sustainable smoky eye

We all love a smokey eye. People avoid this look if, like me, they have smaller, deep-set eyes, but in fact, this look is perfect for you! While technically, yes, a smokey does make your eye appear smaller, but because it's so well defined, visually it gives your eyes deeper definition, which in turn makes them stand out more. You are ideally looking for the colour to appear deepest along your upper and lower lash line, blending out into a lighter colour over the lids and into the socket line. You can have the same colour in different intensities on both the lash line and the lid; you can have one deep colour in the same intensity all over the eye; or you can have one colour on the lid and a different colour lining the lashline. A smokey is a good opportunity to use colours you might have been a bit unsure about using before – greens, purples, navy. Because you will be lining the eye with a darker colour, the intensity of the lid colour is knocked back somewhat, so it makes colour easier to wear. There is a broad spectrum of choices, but the overall look is one of sensuality and intensity.

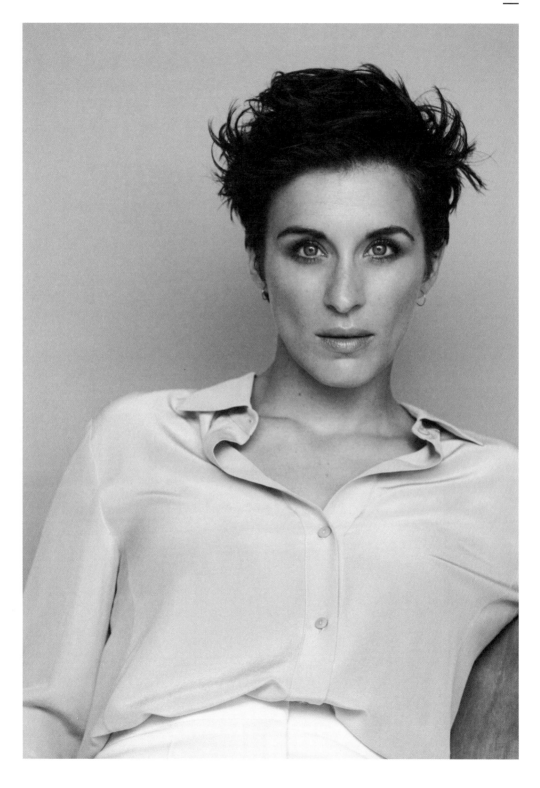

TECHNIQUE: I like to start with a wash of colour over the lids, blended up into the socket line and along the lower lash line. Colours with slight shimmer are more forgiving and easier to blend if you are covering a larger area like the entire surface of the lid. However, a matte colour will give more depth and intensity. A dark taupe, mid or dark brown, or dark grey, are good places to start. You need a brush to lay the colour on and one to buff for a blended edge. Lay the colour on, don't be too precious about it at this stage, and stop at the socket line. Take the buffer brush and using back-and-forth and small circular motions, bring the colour up into the socket line, but don't go too high. Just enough so that, when you look straight ahead, you can see the blended colour just above your socket line. Use a small soft brush to apply and buff into the lower lash line. Don't worry too much about the shape just yet, that can be altered later.

Here is where I like to use a chunky eyeliner crayon. Selecting a darker colour to the one on your lid, place the colour close along the lash line, both upper and lower. Take another small soft blending brush, or your ring finger, and buff the liner so it naturally blurs the definition between shadow and liner. Stand back and check the shape, adjust if you need to, however part of the sexiness of a good smokey eye is that it's not perfect (think Chrissie Hynde or Cara Delevingne). It's a bit smudgy, and a bit worn in. If you want to deepen the intensity, apply a kohl eye pencil or a chunky crayon inside the eye (check first to see if it can be used in the waterline). My eyes are a little close together, so I stop about three-quarters of the way across, leaving the inner corner brighter. This gives the illusion of wider eyes. Don't forget to apply on the upper waterline; this makes your lash line look thicker. Colour combinations I love to use are brown lid/black liner, grey lid/black liner, taupe lid/ dark brown liner, green lid/black liner and purple lid/ dark grey liner.

La Flick

I can't write a book about beauty and not include the eyeliner flick. It's the one thing we all want to master. Your best friends here are your tools. You must have good brushes that are up to the task, or else you'll be forever cleaning up, adjusting, readjusting, taking it all off to start again and pulling your hair out. If you're a make-up artist, a magnifying glass is very useful to check whether you need to make any adjustments. I can't tell you the best brushes to buy, as I think everyone develops their own style of doing an eyeliner flick. What I will say is that once your liner is on, it's not that easy to correct any mistakes, so a finer rather than thicker brush is a good starting point. You can always build up the thickness. Getting the correct shape of the angle is the hardest part, so using a fine line makes it easier to remove or adjust. I like a synthetic brush, obviously, and one that is not going to splay or fray. What I mean by that is that the hair needs to stay flat. If you have even one hair that starts to separate, you'll

struggle to create a straight line, so invest in a good brush. In terms of the liner itself, a gel pot or a cake eyeliner are my preferred options. You may be a total whizz with liquid liner, but they are harder to use and you cannot recycle them so, as far as sustainability goes, they are a no-no. Look for a gel in a reasonably sized glass pot (a pot less than 50mm in diameter is too small to recycle). Cake eyeliners have been around for a long time, but are so useful. If you water them down to a faint line, this is a great way to initially draw on your flick as a guide, and check it without fully committing (using eye shadow also works for this).

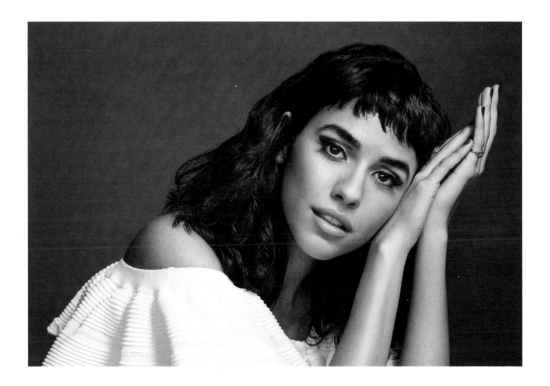

TECHNIQUE: Look straight ahead in a mirror. Place a tiny dot of liner on each eye where you want the flick to end. Stand back and check in a mirror. Do they look roughly symmetrical? Does it give your eye a slight lift? Does it look good? The beauty of just applying the guide dot first is that you can easily make any adjustment. Your eyes are not exactly the same – no one's are, so don't give yourself an impossible task trying to achieve perfect symmetry. An ideal flick angles slightly upwards when looking straight ahead. A flick that angles straight out or downwards can work for a fashion shoot, but for us mere mortals, it'll make our eyes look tired and sad. Once you are happy with your guide dots, look down into a mirror to apply the liner; this way you can see exactly what you're doing, with both eyes open. Looking down also allows you to apply the liner as close to the lash line as possible. It's important to

have zero gaps between lash and liner or it will look patchy. Load the brush, wipe off any excess, and start just a little bit in from the inner corner. The inner corner is where you want the liner to be its thinnest and finest, so you don't want the brush newly loaded with product. Draw the line along the upper lash line until about three-quarters of the way along then stop. Go back and line the inner corner with what's left on the brush. This should give you the finest of lines. Then look straight ahead in the mirror. Reload the brush, remembering to wipe off any excess. Put your ring finger on the outer edge of your brow and gently pull the skin taut and up. Join the end of the liner with the guide dot. You can either start at the liner, meeting the dot, or start at the dot and join to the liner. I do both, depending on what feels right that day.

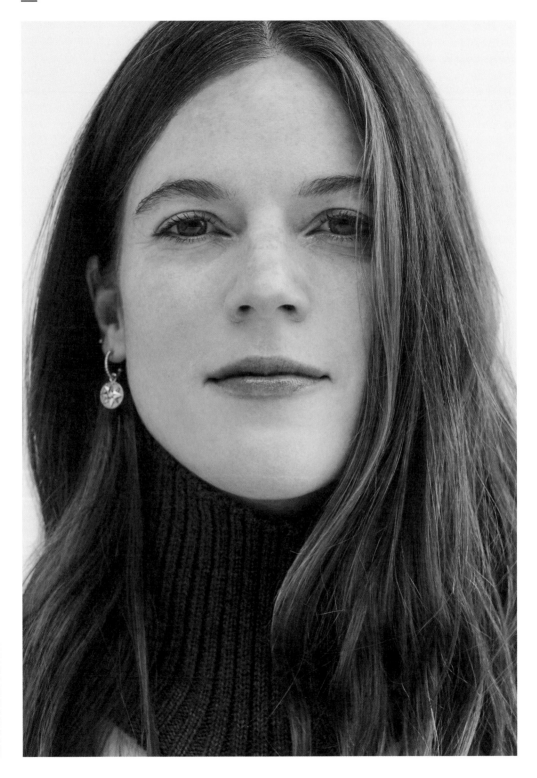

Lips

—

I love lip colour. My personal obsession is red. Vegan red, of course. It's a bold, bright nod to glamour, which makes me feel like me. But red might not be for everyone. Just as well, then, that there are endless shades and textures available, for any skin tone and any age.

It's a fact, though, that we ingest a small amount of anything we put onto our lips. Common ingredients in lip products include refined petroleum, which can generate small amounts of 1,4-dioxane, a substance believed to contribute to some serious health issues. It's not listed as an ingredient as it's a contaminant created when other ingredients react to being mixed together. So, my advice: stick to natural waxes, butters and vegetable oils such as coconut, jojoba and vitamin E.

But we don't need a whole wardrobe of lip colour, so let's think about what we actually use. Most people tend to stick to one product during the day and one product for the evening. So, consider how you like to look. Do you prefer natural colours, bright colours, or a vintage look? Do you like to concentrate on your eyes over your lips? Or are you all about lipstick? Our beauty products must be sustainable. The majority of lip gloss tubes, liquid lipsticks and lipstick bullets require specialist recycling, as they are mixed materials. Only mono materials can be recycled in your recycling bin. They're also not wide enough to be generally recycled. Look up your nearest Terracycle scheme to recycle your lip products. Glass pots of lip colour over 50mm in diameter are a good sustainable option.

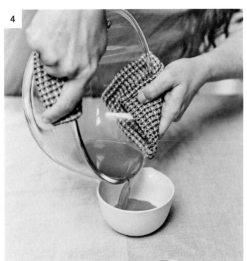

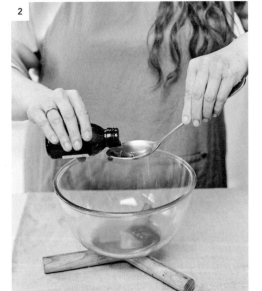

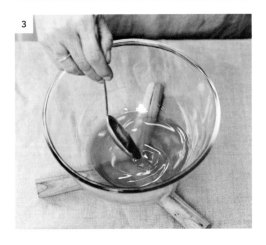

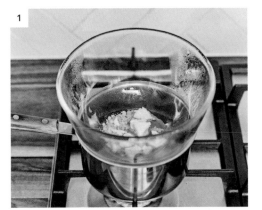

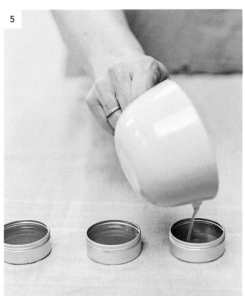

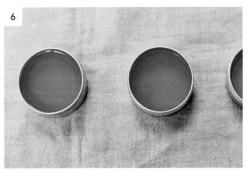

Vegan lip balm

I really like and encourage the multi-use of beauty products. Natural lip balms, such as this vegan one, are fantastic for this. Because they are slightly harder in texture, they are great for also taming brows and fly-away hairs on your head.

Ingredients
–   15g (½oz) jojoba wax
–   15g (½oz) cocoa butter
–   15g (½oz) shea butter
–   2 tbsp jojoba oil
–   4 tsp hemp oil
–   1 tsp vegetable
    glycerine

Equipment
–   Heatproof glass bowl
    that sits snugly on top
    of the saucepan
–   Saucepan
–   Metal spoon
–   Funnel (optional)
–   5 x 15ml (½fl oz) jars or
    tins, sterilised
–   Heatproof jug
–   Heatproof gloves

Method
Fill a saucepan halfway with cold water and bring to the boil. Once boiling, reduce the heat to low, creating a gentle simmer.

1. Place the glass bowl directly on top of the saucepan of simmering water. Add the jojoba wax, cocoa butter and shea butter to the bowl, stirring until they are all melted in together. The water should still be at a simmer; if it starts to boil, take the saucepan off the hob for a few seconds until it's cooled before trying again.

2. Using heat-proof gloves, carefully remove the glass bowl from the saucepan and place on the heatproof surface. Add jojoba oil, hemp oil and glycerine to the mixture.

3. Stir gently with a metal spoon, until everything has combined and is liquid.

4. Pour the hot liquid into the heatproof jug using the funnel, if using.

5–6. Immediately pour the liquid into the sterilised jars to set. Take care, as the mix is extremely hot.

Tip: These also make great gifts.

Lip scrubs and balms

We all occasionally suffer from chapped lips and using a lip scrub will help. Double 'A' face paste is a scrub gentle enough for lips (see page 65), but if they are very sore, massage with a damp muslin cloth in small circular motions instead. Lip balms prevent chapping, as they keep lips soft and hydrated. I use a lot of tinted lip balms to give a hint of colour while still looking natural. They're easy to apply, and as a multi-use product you can also pop a little on the apple of your cheek for that healthy glow. Clear lip balms made from harder waxes are also perfect for taming brows and soothing small patches of dry skin.

Lipstick

Lipsticks are versatile products, usually available in bullet or liquid form. The main ingredients are waxes, oils, emollients (moisturising) and pigments (colour). Textures range from sheer to moisturising to full-on matte. Wear alone or line the lips with lip liner for a sharper shape.

Liquid lipsticks can pack a pigment punch. Thinner in consistency than the bullet, they're applied like a gloss. Their matte formulations do not budge, but can be a bit drying, so apply lip balm first.

TECHNIQUE: For long lasting party lipstick, apply lip liner all over the lips, followed by one coat of a matte or semi-matte formulation. Take one ply of tissue and place over lips. Press setting powder on the tissue, then apply your second coat of lipstick. Lick your lips before sipping a drink and your lipstick will stay on your lips, not on the glass

Liquid lipstick application takes practice, as you don't have much time to correct any mistakes before it dries. Apply to the bottom lip first, then press lips together. Fill in the rest of your lips using a lip brush or the applicator.

Lip liners and crayons

It's all about the texture with a lip liner. Harder pencils will produce sharper lines and softer textures will create a more diffused line. Filling in the entire lip with lip pencil gives your lipstick more staying power, but use a soft pencil otherwise it'll take too long and you'll make your lips sore in the process. If you want to wear a bright lipstick and lip liner, but you're lacking in confidence, apply your lipstick first leaving the edges clear, then apply your liner after. The lipstick acts as a guideline for the lip liner.

Lip crayons are a fabulous two-in-one product. They are available in different textures, from gloss to matte. My only gripe is you need to sharpen them often. Apart from that, they are a joy to use, as they are easy to apply and you do not need a separate lip liner.

Lip gloss

Gloss can be worn alone or over another lip colour. Be prepared for touch-ups throughout the day as they're not as long-lasting as lipstick. For natural formulations, look for oils like coconut, jojoba and vitamin E. If you have fine lines around your lips, avoid colour glosses, as this product will bleed more easily. If you want the glossy look, but have fine lines, use a clear gloss alone. Alternatively, line and fill the lips with a coloured lip pencil, and apply clear gloss on top.

Lip stains

Stains are long-lasting liquids that come in a bottle or as a pen, and give a lovely, natural matte hue. They can also multitask as cheek stains. If using an alcohol-based stain, which can by drying, use a lip balm first.

Lip and cheek tints

These multitaskers come in various formulations including liquids, creams and gels, in sticks, pots and tubes. Choose tints with balm textures created from natural coconut oil, waxes and butters for a soft, natural make up.

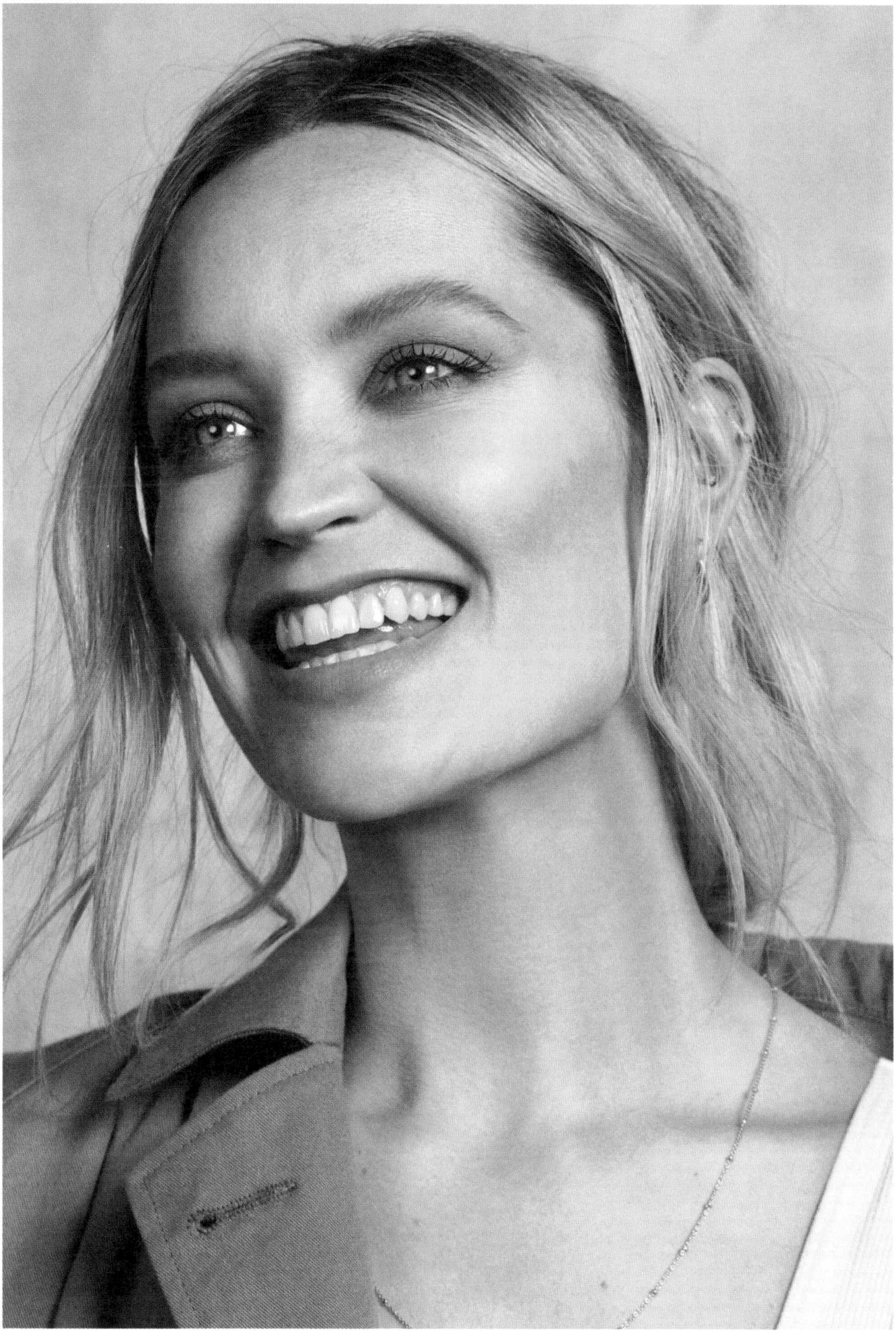

The mindful make-up tool kit

—

If you're passionate about beauty, it's impossible not to be seduced by new brands, colours, textures and packaging. If you believe everything brands tell you, you'll collect a drawer full of products that would even confuse the Kardashians, and a holographic glittery eyeshadow that you'll only use at a festival once. While it's fun to have the odd specialist product or colour, our over-consumption is having catastrophic effects on our planet. If you have fewer, more carefully chosen products in your make-up kit, everything has breathing space. You'll feel more organised and the act of applying make-up becomes ritualised and joyful, rather than a rummage, a rush and a frenzy.

The perfect make-up kit

The following is a checklist of the type and number of products typically in your make-up bag, together with ideas for easy sustainable swaps.

Biodegradable blotting papers – absorb any excess oil.

Blusher (2) – in powder, cream or liquid formulations. Try using your moisturising lipstick as a cream blusher and vice versa (matte textures will be hard to blend).

Eyelash curlers (1) – these really do give that va-va-voom to your lashes. If you choose a mascara with a lifting formulation, you won't need curlers.

Eyeshadow palette (1) – a basic palette of nude shadows (including cream, taupe, grey, chocolate brown) in both matt and shimmer textures will see you far, plus a matt black to soften the edges of eyeliner.

Eyeliner (3) – black, brown and grey is all you really need, plus a flesh colour for inside the waterline if you often have red eyes.

Bronzer (1) – stick to a powder formulation.

Contour (1) – for some, a separate contour product is essential. If that is not you, then use your bronzer to cut down on products.

Highlighter (1) – for a natural look, avoid a highly mirrored-finish highlighter. To save on products, use a shimmer eyeshadow as a highlighter instead.

Eyebrow pencil/balm (1) – for those that prefer a natural brow, you can swap out this product and use an eyeshadow applied with an angled brush.

Lip balm (2) – can also be used to tame brow hairs and as a natural highlight on cheekbones.

Lip liner (2) – can be used all over the lips with lip balm as your lip colour or switch to a lip crayon, which acts as a two-in-one lipstick and lip liner.

Day lip colour (2) – try using as a cream blusher.

Evening lip colour (2) – try using as a cream blusher.

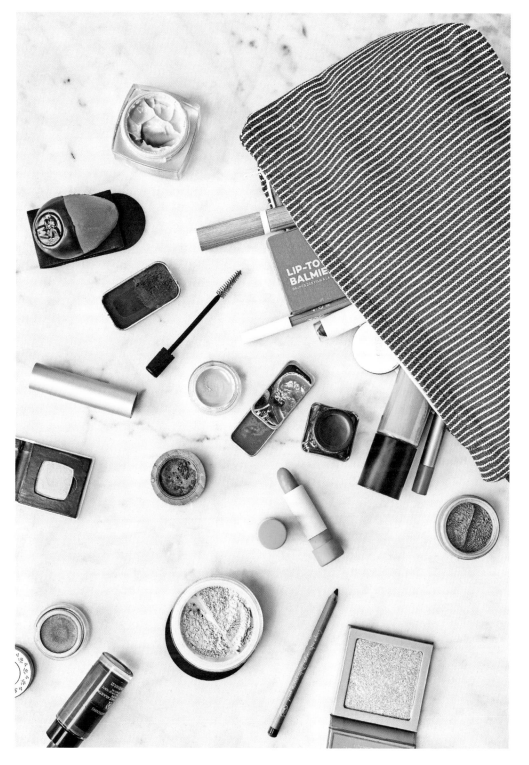

The essential tool kit

There are a plethora of make-up tools out there, with brands telling you that this tool will change your life, improve your make-up and be the next big thing. From gua sha facial massage tools to beauty blenders to cleansing brushes, there's a lot of products on the market. Here's a rundown of what you actually need.

Make-up brushes

A staple for anyone that likes to wear make-up. Invest in a good-quality set, take care of them and they should last you for many years. Always buy vegan make-up brushes, even if you're not vegan. Many people will claim vegan brushes don't pick up and apply the product as well, but I can attest to the fact that they do. Technology with synthetic hair has come on leaps and bounds, plus it's more hygienic and prevents cruelty to animals. There is an argument that the production of synthetic hair uses more resources to make. That's impossible to know, as you'd have to contact each individual factory to assess their methods, but nothing is worth the torture of animals in my book. Vegan brushes all the way.

Brush cleaning

Cleaning your make-up brushes is vital for your skin health. They harbour bacteria, dirt and grime. Cleanse them like you would your hair, with a couple of drops of tea tree oil added in for antibacterial benefits. If you are allergic to tea tree oil or have highly sensitive skin, cleanse with a co-wash or shampoo, condition, and leave to dry on a towel. If you can, avoid placing the brushes on a flat surface as they will dry with an odd shape. Leave them hanging over the edge of a sink. Try not to get the ferrule (the aluminium middle section) wet and you will prolong the life of your brushes. There are now a few brush-cleaning driers and spinning machines on the market, like the StylPro.

Eyelash curlers

If you have straight eyelashes, then invest in a good pair of lash curlers. Don't bother with cheap versions; they won't work. If your budget doesn't allow, choose a mascara with lifting technology. Never use them without the rubber lining, and don't use curlers every day, or else you will weaken your lashes. Avoid curling once you have applied mascara (a very gentle curl if you must) or your lashes will stick to the curlers. When the rubber lining starts to perish, replace it.

Tweezers

These incredibly useful items are something you'd be wise to invest in. All you'll ever really need is a slant tweezer. This style sits comfortably in your hand and can also be used to apply false lashes. When tweezing facial hair, if you pull the skin tight (gently), it won't hurt quite as much.

Sharpener

I'm *very* particular about my pencil sharpeners. Invest in one with a good-quality razor to keep your pencils sharp and smooth and a container to catch the shavings in case you are nowhere near a bin. The best one I've found so far is made by My Kit Co. If you have motor difficulties, then invest in a good-quality electric sharpener.

Nail kit

You just need clippers, scissors, a glass file and a couple of orange sticks to keep your nails groomed and your cuticles hydrated.

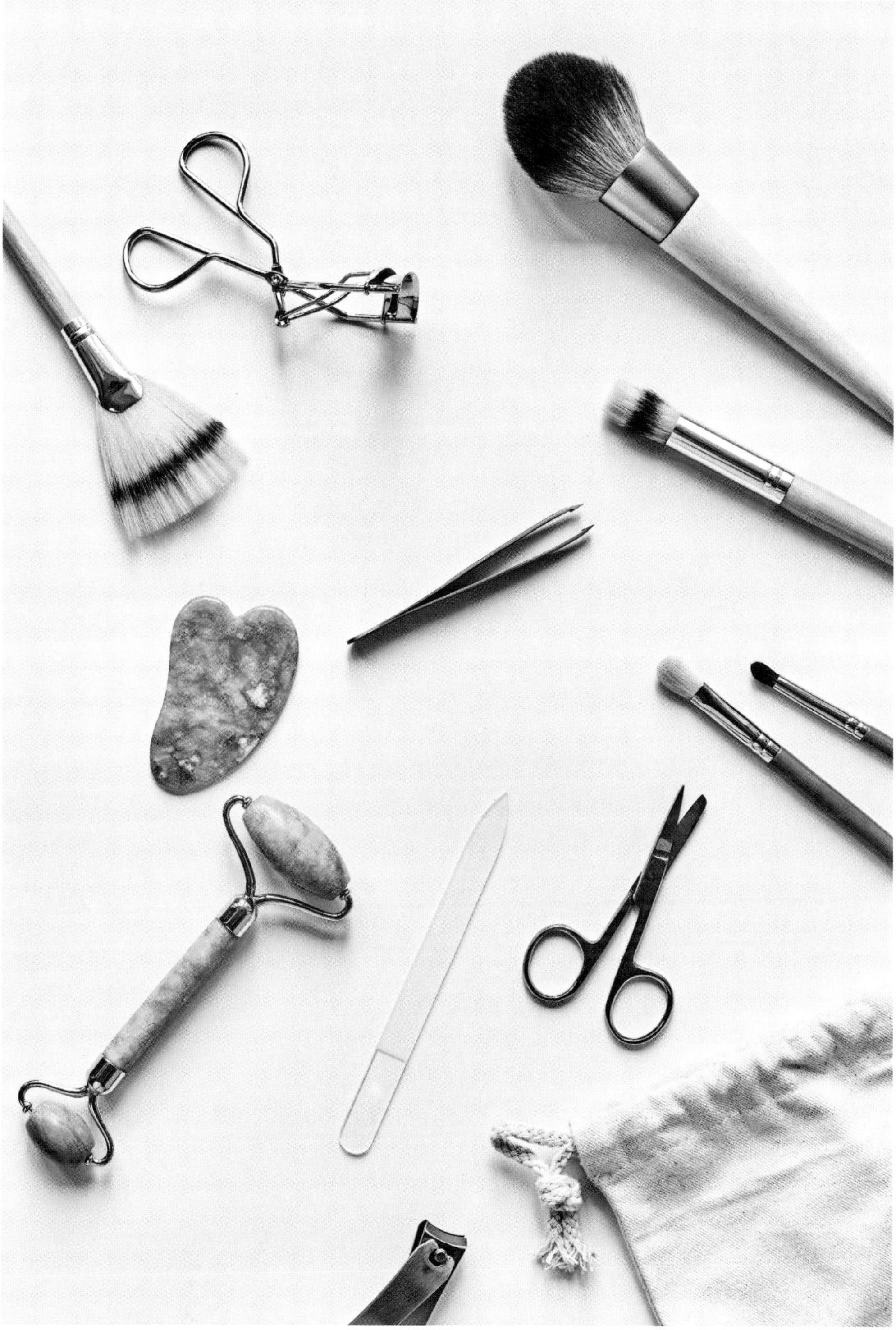

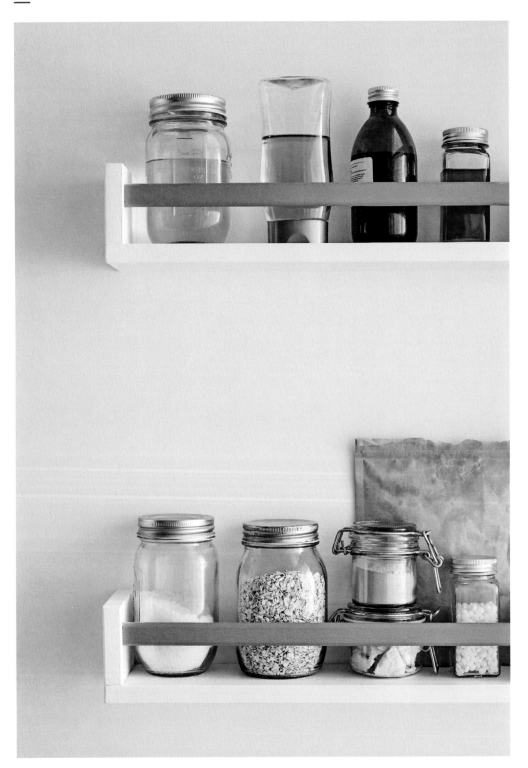

Beauty Larder

—

As you become familiar with making your own beauty products, you'll start to build a larder of ingredients that can form the base from everything from a body scrub to a lip balm. Start small, with a handful of items and slowly add to your collection as you become more adept at making products. Select cold pressed oils where possible as they are extracted using mechanical methods as opposed to using solvents. The ingredients you choose will depend on your skin type and preferred scents but here are some of the multi-purpose products that make up my beauty larder.

- apple cider vinegar (raw)
- aloe vera (10:1 concentrate)
- agave
- argan oil
- arrowroot powder
- avocado
- baking powder
- borage oil
- castor oil
- cedarwood essential oil
- CBD oil
- cinnamon powder
- clary sage oil
- clove powder
- cocoa butter (unrefined)
- coconut oil
- fractionated coconut oil
- virgin unrefined coconut oil
- cucumber
- ethyl alcohol (food grade)
- Epsom salts
- frankincense essential oil
- green clay
- green tea
- hemp oil
- jojoba oil
- lavender essential oil
- dried lavender flowers
- lemon juice
- mandarin essential oil
- oats (organic)
- olive oil
- peppermint essential oil
- pumpkin seed oil
- rose essential oil
- rose water
- rosehip seed oil
- rosemary essential oil
- sandalwood oil
- sea salt
- shea butter (unrefined)
- sweet almond oil
- tea tree essential oil
- vegetable glycerine
- vitamin E oil
- vervain essential oil
- vetiver essential oil
- witch hazel
- ylang ylang essential oil
- zinc oxide

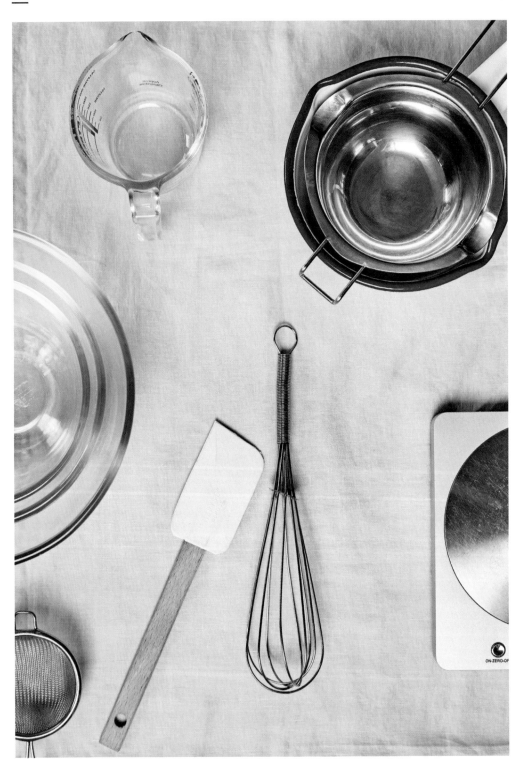

Beauty Tool Shed

—

One of the wonderful things about making your own beauty items is that you don't require any special equipment. A few standard items from your kitchen cupboards is all you need to make a whole range of products. Below is my tried and tested tool shed which will allow you to make all of the recipes in this book.

- Blender or food processor
- Dropper bottles (repurposed)
- Electric or handheld whisk
- Face cloth
- Glass atomizer bottles (repurposed)
- Glass jars with lids of various sizes (repurposed)
- Glass pump bottles (repurposed)
- Hair net or hair covering
- Heatproof gloves
- Heatproof pouring jug
- Heatproof glass bowls of various sizes
- Heatproof measuring beakers
- Metal fork
- Metal spoon
- Mixing bowl
- Muslin (cheesecloth) square
- Nitrile disposable gloves
- Rubber band or hair band (repurposed)
- Saucepans
- Scales
- Small aluminium tins (repurposed)
- Spatula
- Twine or repurposed white or cream ribbon (dye can be released from wet coloured ribbon)

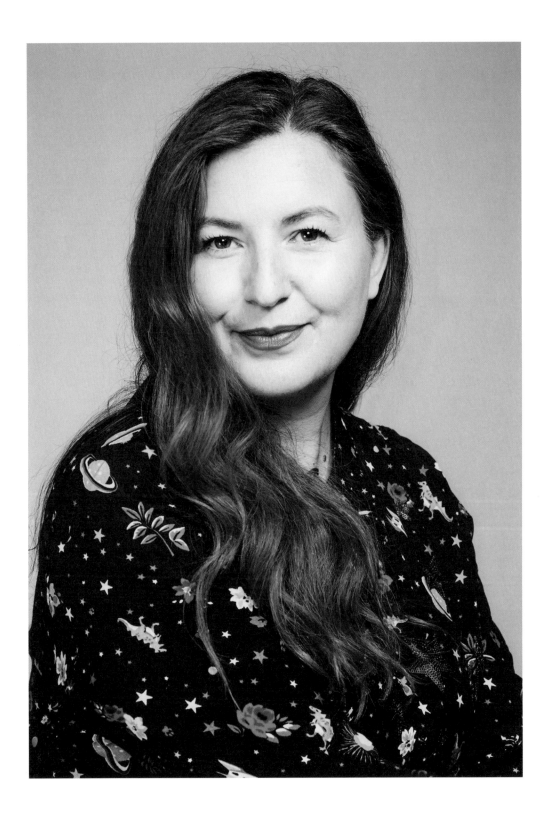

Conclusion

—

The power of make up and beauty is magical, and its transformational power can lift our spirits and elevate our self esteem. Like moths to moonlight, we are intensely attracted to the luminosity and light of cosmetics and beauty. However, where there is light there is shadow. The business of beauty is huge. In the UK alone, the beauty industry was worth a whopping £28.4 billion in 2018. While this indicates a thriving industry, this insatiable appetite for beauty has consequences. If only we had heeded the advice of indigenous communities the world over to 'tread lightly upon the earth.' We didn't. And now we, and the planet, are paying the price.

How we got here, will inform how we change. So let's look at how big brands operate. Large corporations have a legal duty to their shareholders, so they have to maximise profits *at all costs*. As a result the corporation is almost pathological in nature wielding huge power over people and societies. Within their need to maximise profits is where we, the consumer can effect change, and where the solution lies. The power of choice reflected in our spending is mighty! It is a barometer of our values, conscience and ethics. This power has force, and can reveal both to brands and the wider beauty industry the direction of our moral compass. If we lead, they will follow. So lead, we must.

Interest in sustainability has to convert into actionable results. There is a large gap between the number of consumers who say they are interested in sustainable products and the number of consumers who actually purchase them. It could be lack of brand transparency, loyalty to brands we already use, or simply that being sustainable is not very convenient. We need to shift our mindset. The issues of human rights, deforestation, environmental damage, diversity and animal rights need to become more important than convenience, and how good a product makes us look or feel. The biggest shift will come when you have your own light bulb moment, that what one buys and uses directly affects our environment and each other. Perhaps a sentence in this book has sparked that connection, or maybe that will come through your own personal journey.

Brands, both large and small also need to step up to the challenge. Big brands have the power and the funding for innovation and to improve the entire infrastructure of the beauty industry to move towards more sustainability. They are making inroads, but due to their size, changes take longer to implement. The smaller indie brands have more flexibility and can build new business models shifting away from a focus purely on profit. They are ingenious with product ideas and development, however they don't necessarily have the financial clout nor the power to affect decisions at the top of the industry pyramid. I believe the beauty industry has the opportunity to be a beacon for other industries to follow. Brands need to share knowledge and join together to create and new more sustainable future for beauty.

I hope this book has inspired you to look behind the veil of glitzy packaging and glamorous marketing. To be more conscious, to think about and research what products you are buying, how you are using them and what happens to them at the end of their life. We can all reduce. We consumers can cut down on what we use and buy and brands can focus on quality and ethics, as opposed to endless product launches. I'm not perfect. I still use products in my professional kit that don't tick all the sustainable boxes. Simply because otherwise I wouldn't be able to do my job to the best of my abilities. Some of my favourite brands have a strong focus on clean and organically grown ingredients that support communities, but their packaging isn't easily recyclable, or they are vegan but the ingredients are synthetic. So do not feel that because you haven't ethically overhauled your entire make up bag and bathroom cabinet, that you're not making a difference. You are. If we join together and support sustainable beauty as much as we can, and as best we can, then we can be excited to see what the future of the beauty industry holds. Let's create a consumer led sustainable beauty revolution, before it's too late. Power to the people!

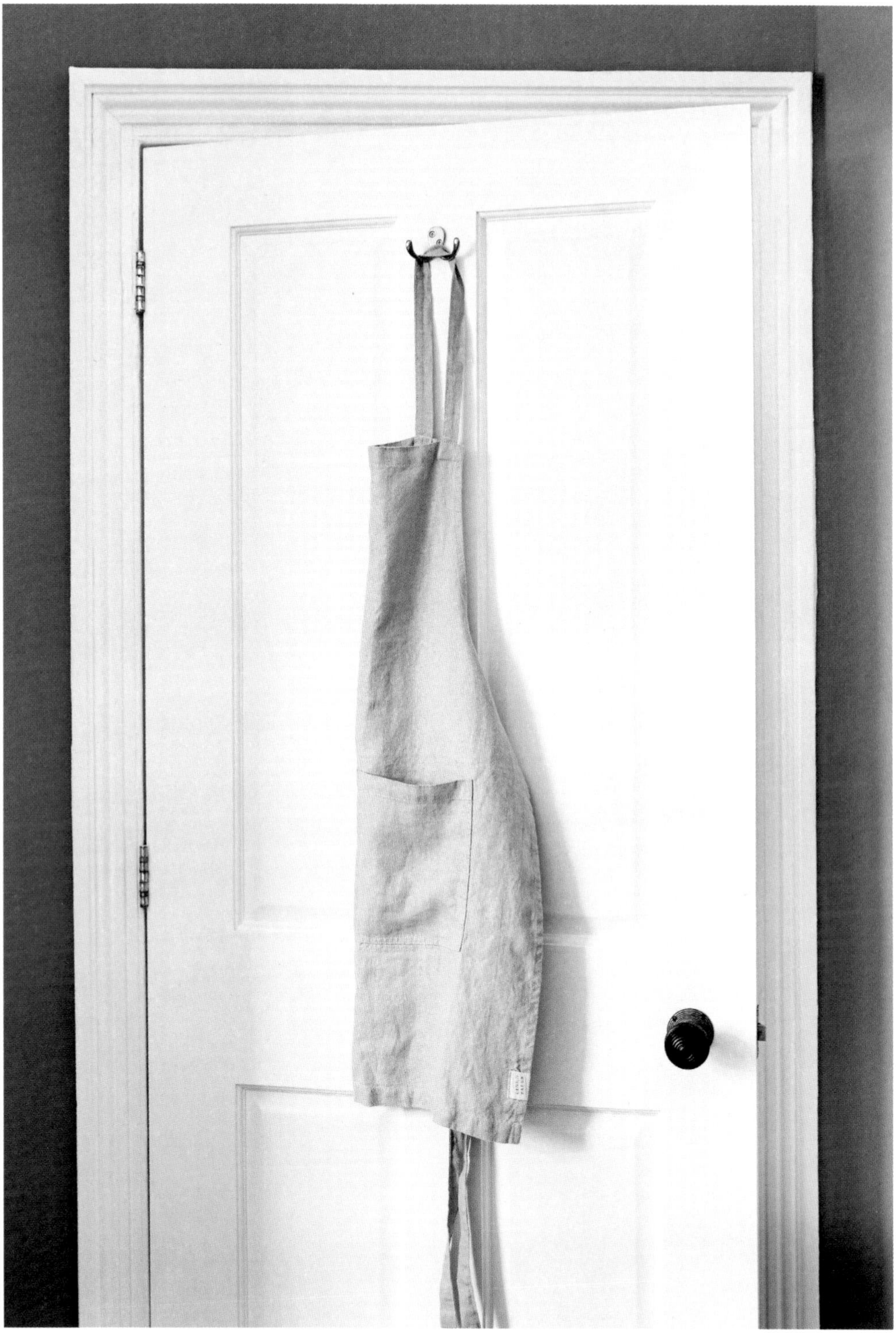

Animal-derived ingredients
—

The following list of animal-derived products may also help in your buying choices. I have given alternative vegan choices, which are marked VA, meaning Vegan Alternative.

Allantoin – uric acid from mammals, used mainly in creams and lotions.

Ambergris – derived from the waxy oil that lines whale's stomachs. Used in perfumes.

Animal collagen – the fibrous protein from animal tissue, found in lip-plumping products and skincare. VA: soya protein, almond oil.

Beeswax (cera alba) – used as an emulsifier, gives structure to formulae by keeping emulsions from separating into oil and liquid. Found in many cosmetics and skincare products. VA: synthetic beeswax, plant and soya waxes.

Carmine (cochineal dye) – a red dye obtained by crushing tens of thousands of female cochineal beetles (*Dactylopius coccus*) to make a small amount of dye. Carmine is found in most non-vegan red lipsticks, blushers and other red-coloured make-up. Also known as natural red 4, E120, C.I.75470.

Casein – derived from cow's milk and used in hair products and skincare. VA: plant-based milks, labelled as vegetable protein.

Caprylic acid – a fatty acid found in animal milk. It's an antimicrobial and antifungal agent, used as a preservative. Also known as caprylyl glycol. VA: flower and bark extracts which can also be listed as caprylic acid, so if it's not clear, contact the brand.

Cholestoral – a fatty acid derived from animal fats, used as an emulsifier. Also known as C10-30 cholesterol/lanosterol esters. VA: plant-derived fatty acids.

Elastin – extracted from the muscles, ligaments and aortas of animals. Found in lip-pumping products and skincare. VA: hyaluronic acid and MSM.

Gelatin – made from the boiled bones, skin, tendons and ligaments of animals; found in creamy cosmetics.

Glycerine – generally comes from animal fats and is used in soaps, hair products, make-up and skincare as a softener. Also known as ethylhexylglycerin, glycerides, glyceryls, glycreth-26, polyglycerol. VA: alternative vegetable glycerin (is sometimes just marked as glycerine so look for vegan certification or contact the brand).

Guanine – crushed fish scales used to create shimmer and light-diffusing properties. Found in highlighters, sparkly nail polish, eyeshadow, bronzers and blushers.

Hyaluronic acid – can be derived from animals or plants. Used to hydrate; helps skin retain water. Also known as sodium hyaluronate, glycosaminoglycan, hyaluran, hyaluronan, hyaluronate sodium, hylan. If it's not clear that the hyaluronic acid is plant-based, contact the brand.

Keratin – derived from the hair and horns of animals. Found in nail and hair products. VA: Soya protein and almond oil.

Lanolin (wool grease) – an emollient derived from wool-bearing animals and is found in many lip products and some hair products. Used to soften and moisturise. Also known as acetylated lanolin oil or wax.

Lecithin – derived from animal or plant sources. If vegan, it will usually be labelled as 'soy lecithin'. Used as a skin softener and soother. VA: plant oils.

Isopropyl Lanolate, Aliphatic Alcohols, Cholesterin, Lanolin Alcohols, Lanosterols, Sterols, Triterpene Alcohols. VA plant oils and butters.

Oestrogen (estradiol) – extracted from the urine of pregnant horses. Used in perfumes and skincare.

Retinol – a potent source of vitamin A and is almost always derived from an animal, unless the product is vegan. It's used to condition and soften the skin. Also known as retinol acetate, retinyl palmitate and vitamin A.

Shellac – resinous product from lac insects used in nail products and hairsprays.

Squalene – extracted from shark-liver oil. Found in eye make-up, lip products, deodorants and skincare. VA: vegan squalene derived from plant-seed oils, olives and wheat germ. Also known as shark liver oil, squalane.

Stearic acid – generally derived from pigs' stomachs but can also come from cows, sheep and cats in laboratories. Found in deodorant, soap, hair products and moisturisers. Also listed as isostearyl neopentanoate, stearamide, stearamine, stearates, stearic hydrazide, stearone, stearoxytrimethylsilane, stearoyl lactylic acid, stearyl betaine, stearyl imidazoline, sorbitan sesquioleate. Can also be listed as stearic acid even if plant based, so contact the brand if it's not clear. VA: plant fats and natural minerals.

Tallow (oleic acid) – an animal fat obtained by boiling the carcasses of slaughtered animals until a fatty substance is produced. It is added to many make-up products, including soap, foundations, nail polishes, eye make-up and lip products. VA: can be derived from plant sources such as coconut, olives and nuts.

Index

—

A

acetone 20

AHA 20

air drying hair 97

alcohol in cosmetics 20

alcohol free products 18

aluminium 36–37

animal derived ingredients 154–155

animal testing 27

antiperspirants 73

arrowroot deodorant cream 74–75

B

balm, magic all-purpose rescue balm 70–71

beauty industry 6–8

BHA 20

biodegradable products 32

biodynamic skincare 18

bismuth oxychloride 20

blue beauty 18

blushers 124–125

Body Shop 6

bodycare 73

    arrowroot deodorant cream 74–75

    bedtime pillow bliss mist 104

    body lotions, creams, butters and oils 80

    body washes and scrubs 73, 78–79

    dry brushing 80

    hands, feet and nails 84–89

    JJ's miracle moon oil for period pains 106–107

    oat soak for sensitive skin 76–77

    rose soufflé body butter for dry skin 82–83

    spiced tooth powder 108

bronzers 124

brows 127–128

C

carbon neutral products 18

CBD skincare 18

chemical free products 18

clean beauty 18

cleansing 49–52

jojoba facial cleansing oil 50–51

co-washing conditioners 91

compostable products 32

concealers 118, 129

conditioners 91–92

conscious consumption 11–12

contouring 120

cosmetic ingredients 20–21, 103

Cruelty Free International (CFI) 25

cruelty-free beauty 25–29

curl creams 98

D

deodorants 73, 74–75

dermatologically tested 18

dry brushing 80

dry shampoo 91

E

Ellen MacArthur Foundation 31

essential oils 20

ethical buying 23

    animal testing 27

    cruelty-free beauty 25

    ethical brands 27

    parent companies 29

    sourcing your product 24–25

    vegan and vegetarian beauty 28

eye cream 62

eye make-up 126

    brows 127–128

    concealer 129

    essential eye kit 130

    eye make-up techniques 132–135

    eye shadow 130

    mascara 129

eye patches 62

F

face masks 64–67, 68

face powder 119

facial cleansing brushes 52

facial mists/spritzes 55, 58–9

facial oils 62

facial scrubs 54–55

feet 84

rosemary and tea tree foot soak 88–89

foundation 115–116

    application techniques 118

fragrance 20

free radicals 21

G

glass 37

Greenpeace 19, 24, 25, 35

H

haircare 90

    hair cleansing 91

    hair healing rinse 100–101

    hair masks 92, 94-95

    hair nourishing 91–92

    hairspray 98

    heat protection products 98

    ingredients to be aware of 103

    styling 97

    styling products 97–98

hands 84

    vodka and grapefruit hand sanitizer 86–87

hemp towels 97

highlighting 121–122

homemade products 44

    bain marie use 46–47

    beauty larder 146

    beauty tool shed 148

    melting coconut oil 47

    practical tips 46

    prepping your area 47

    sterilising jars and bottles 47

    why make your own beauty products? 44–46

hypoallergenic products 18

I

INCI (International Nomenclature of Cosmetic Ingredients) 17

ingredients 20–21, 103

    animal derived ingredients 154–155

Instagram 7, 8, 11, 115, 116, 120

J
jojoba facial cleansing oil 50–51
Juni Cosmetics 37

L
labels 17
    ingredients 20–21, 103
    terminology 17–19
Leaping Bunny 25
leave-in hair treatments 92
lips 137
    lip and cheek tints 141
    lip gloss 141
    lip liners and crayons 141
    lip scrubs and balms 140
    lip stains 141
    lipstick 140
    vegan lip balm 138–139
Logical Harmony 27
Loop 25, 36

M
magnets 37
make-up 111–112
    blusher and bronzer 124–125
    contour and highlight 120–122
    eye make-up 126–135
    foundation, concealer and powder 115–119
    lips 137–141
make-up kit 142–143
    essential tool kit 144–145
mascara 129
Mexican hair mask 94–95
mica 24
microbiome skincare 18–19
microplastics 37
Milady's Skin Care and Cosmetics Ingredients Dictionary 17
miscellar waters 52
moisturiser 63

N
nails 84
natural skincare 19
night time body scrubs 78–79

non-comogenic products 19
non-GMO products 19
non-toxic products 19

O
oat face mask 66–67
oat soak for sensitive skin 76–77
organic products 19

P
packaging 31
    magnets 37
    microplastics 37
    outer and inner packaging 37
    plastic packaging 34–35
    recyclable, biodegradable and compostable 32
    refillable beauty 35–36
    repurposing packaging 38, 47
    specialist recycling 35
    sustainable packaging options 36–37
palm oil 24–25
paraben-free products 19
parent companies 29
period pains, miracle moon oil for 106–107
pillow mists 104
plastic packaging 31, 34–37
propellants 21, 103

R
recyclable products 32
recycling 32, 35
root lift 97
rose soufflé body butter for dry skin 82–83
rosemary and tea tree foot soak 88–89

S
serums 55
    face serum for all skin types 60–61
setting lotions 97–98
shampoos 91
silicones 21, 103

skincare 48
    cleansing 49–52
    double 'A' face paste 64–65
    essential skin care list 68
    eye cream 62
    eye patches 62
    facial masks and sheet masks 68
    facial mists/spritzes 55
    facial oils 62
    facial scrubs 54–55
    magic all-purpose rescue balm 70–71
    moisturiser 63
    oat face mask 66–67
    serums 55, 60–61
    skin elixir for all ages 56–57
    spot treatment 68
    spritz of rosewater, cucumber & green tea 58–9
    toning 53–54
slow beauty 19
sourcing your product 24–25
spots 118
    spot treatment 68
styling mousses and gels 97
surfactants 21, 103
sustainable beauty 15, 41, 151–152
    homemade products 44–47
sustainable products 19

T
TerraCycle 23, 35, 36, 47
toners 53–54
tooth powder, spiced 108

V
vegan and vegetarian beauty 28
    vegan lip balm 138–139
    animal derived ingredient substitutes 154–155
vodka and grapefruit hand sanitizer 86–87

W–Z
wipes 52
zero waste products 19

Acknowledgements

—

I am grateful to many people who have been part of writing this book and supporting my work. To Zara Anvari, Jessica Axe and Charlotte Frost, I extend my gratitude for leading the way into this project and for their skill, hard work and frightening efficiency. To the creative director, Rachel Cross, for having and holding such an elegant vision. To our photographer, Emma Guscott, who beautifully captured the energy. To Amanda Harris, for her expertise and guidance. I extend heartful gratitude to my partner Lee Smith, to my sister, Nancy Jenkins and my PA Michelle Crease, for their valuable support and involvement in this project and their belief in me. I couldn't have done it without you.

My love and gratitude to Jean and Tony – mum and dad, for your constant support and love. Treasures in my life. To my nephew Max, our heart, and a shining light to us all. To Honey, Alice and Lucas. To Nic, Mart, Shep, Jo H and Rebecca R. To my family, I love you all. To my five adopted and beloved fur-babies: Sonny, Wanda, Tippi, Velma and Teddy-Dumpling. Their comedy capers and unending joy kept me going on long nights of writing. Not forgetting my past fur loves Frodo and Maggie, my spirit guides. Thank you to Wendy Higgins and Humane Society International for your tireless work to protect animals and for having me as your beauty ambassador. To all the abused laboratory, farmed, domesticated and wild animals whom I will fight for until my last breath.

Thank you to the friends and colleagues who kindly allowed me to use our work together in this book: Alexa Pearson, Alicia Rountree, Anya Chalotra, Billie Scheepers, Eleanor Tomlinson, Emily Beecham, Fearne Cotton, Fenton Bailey, Gertie Lowe, Jon Gorrigan, Josh Shinner, Keeley Hawes, Laura Whitmore, Rachell Smith, Rose Leslie, Simon Jones, Stephanie Sian Smith, Tim Beaumont, Vicky McLure, Victoria Lennox and Victoria Raeburn Wales.

I'm extremely blessed to have friends who I both love and admire. You have all supported and enriched the writing of this book. Two of whom, in this particular context have been my wise women. Those who have trod the literary track before. They both have for years encouraged me to write. And when I did, they believed in me from the beginning and encouraged me through the writing process. Thank you, Fearne Cotton and Kelly Hoppen, you rock! To all my women folk, you are my heart. The women I've loved and lost, my inspirations: my grandmothers Lillian and Nell, Carol, Ellen, Eve and Saima.

There would be no book, no cause, no career without my fabulous clients, you know who you are. I adore my work and that is because of the people. It is always because of the people. I couldn't wish to work with more uniquely creative, brilliant, kind and good people. It's everything and I relish that I have opportunity to thank them in this way. Also, thank you to all the publicists, photographers, hair stylists, stylists, editors, fashion, photo and creative directors for being my wonderful work family.
I feel it also my duty to thank with open heart all of the brands whose ethics are aimed high, whose hearts are open to concepts and methods of production which preserve and sustain the planet and its peoples; whose profits are earned with integrity and compassion. And who treat and dialogue with their customers as friends.

And with that I thank you. Not just the reader. The human being with this book (or tablet) in their hands. Thank you for supporting sustainability and for making a difference.

First published in 2021 by White Lion Publishing
an imprint of The Quarto Group.
The Old Brewery, 6 Blundell Street
London, N7 9BH, United Kingdom
T (0)20 7700 6700
www.QuartoKnows.com

A catalogue record for this book is available from the British Library.

ISBN 978-0-7112-6597-4
Ebook ISBN 978-0-7112-6599-8

10 9 8 7 6 5 4 3 2 1

Design by Rachel Cross

Printed in China

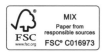

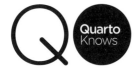

Brimming with creative inspiration, how-to projects and useful information to enrich your everyday life, Quarto Knows is a favourite destination for those pursuing their interests and passions. Visit our site and dig deeper with our books into your area of interest: Quarto Creates, Quarto Cooks, Quarto Homes, Quarto Lives, Quarto Drives, Quarto Explores, Quarto Gifts, or Quarto Kids.